peaceful places
Boston

Other titles of interest

Peaceful Places: Chicago

Peaceful Places: Los Angeles

Peaceful Places: New York City

Peaceful Places: San Francisco

peaceful places
Boston

121 Tranquil Sites in
the City and Beyond

by Lynn Schweikart

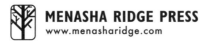

MENASHA RIDGE PRESS
www.menasharidge.com

Peaceful Places: Boston

Copyright © 2012 by Lynn Schweikart
All rights reserved
Published by Menasha Ridge Press
Printed in the United States of America
Distributed by Publishers Group West
First edition, first printing

Cover design by Scott McGrew
Text design by Annie Long
Cartography by Steve Jones
Unless otherwise noted, all cover, back cover, and interior photographs by Lynn Schweikart
Back cover, center photograph: © Thomas Lingner, 2008. *Back cover, right photograph:* Japan: Buddhist Temple Room at the Museum of Fine Arts, Boston; photograph © Museum of Fine Arts, Boston
Cover: For a peaceful time to visit Swan Boats of Boston at the Public Garden, see page 239.

Library of Congress Cataloging-in-Publication Data

    Schweikart, Lynn.
        Peaceful places, Boston : 120 tranquil sites in the city and beyond / Lynn Schweikart.
           p. cm. — (Peaceful places)
        ISBN-13: 978-0-89732-542-4 (pbk.)
        ISBN-10: 0-89732-542-7 ()
        1. Boston (Mass.)—Guidebooks. 2. Quietude. I. Title.
        F869.M394S38 2011
        917.44'610444—dc23
                          2011041986

Menasha Ridge Press
P.O. Box 43673
Birmingham, Alabama 35243
menasharidge.com

Disclaimer

Seclusion can be part of the charm of a peaceful place. Likewise, in some locations, the best time to visit is early morning, sunset, or even in the evening, when few other people are around. Therefore, we remind you to maintain awareness and practice caution in all of the destinations described in this book just as you would when venturing to any isolated or unfamiliar location.

    Also, every effort has been made to ensure the accuracy of information throughout this book, and the contents of this publication are believed to be correct at the time of printing. Nevertheless, the publishers cannot accept responsibility for errors or omissions, for changes in details given in this guide, or for the consequences of any reliance on the information provided by the same. Assessments of sites are based on the author's own experience; therefore, descriptions given in this guide necessarily contain an element of subjective opinion, which may not reflect the publisher's opinion or dictate a reader's own experience on another occasion.

contents

Dedication. x
Acknowledgments xi
Introduction xiii
Three Paths to 121 Peaceful Places xv
Peaceful Places by Category xviii
Peaceful Places by Area. xxiii
Maps xxviii
Peaceful Places Alphanumerically (page numbers listed below) 1
About the Author 262

peaceful places alphanumerically

1   Addison Gallery of American Art 1
2   Allandale Farm and Roadside Stand 4
3   Arlington Street Church 6
4   Arnold Arboretum of Harvard University 8

5   B&G Oysters 11
6   Bates Hall, Boston Public Library 13
7   Beacon Hill Stroll 15
8   Belle Isle Marsh Reservation 18
9   Boston Athenæum 20
10 Boston Common, Frog Pond Skating 23
11 Boston Harbor Islands National Park 25
12 Boston HarborWalk, Downtown to North End 27
13 Boston Marine Society and Shipyard Park 30
14 Boston Nature Center and Wildlife Sanctuary 32
15 Boston Public Library Courtyard. 34

16 Cafe 939, Berklee School of Music 36
17 Cambridge Center Garage Roof Garden 38
18 Charles River Gondola Ride. 40

19 Charles River Kayaking 43
20 Chinatown Park 46
21 Christian Science Center Reflecting Pool 48
22 City Square Park 50
23 Codman Estate 52
24 Commonwealth Avenue Mall 54
25 Condor Street Urban Wild 57
26 Copley Plaza Hotel Oak Room 59
27 Copley Square Farmers' Market 61

28 D. Blakely Hoar Sanctuary 63
29 deCordova Sculpture Park and Museum 65
30 Dorchester Heights 68

31 L'Espalier Salon 70
32 Ether Dome, Massachusetts General Hospital 72

33 Faneuil Hall 74
34 Fenway Park 76
35 Fenway Victory Gardens 79
36 Forest Hills Cemetery 81
37 470 Atlantic Avenue Observation Deck 84
38 Franklin Square 86
39 French Cultural Center of Boston 88
40 Fruitlands Museum 90

41 Gloucester Street Dock 93
42 Greater Boston Buddhist Cultural Center 95
43 Gropius House 97
44 Guest House at Field Farm 99
45 Guild of Boston Artists 102

46 Habitat Education Center and Wildlife Sanctuary 104
47 Hall's Pond Sanctuary and Amory Woods 106

48 Harvard Divinity School Quadrangle Labyrinth 108
49 Harvard Museum of Natural History and Peabody Museum of
Archaeology and Ethnology 110
50 Harvard Square Bookstores 112
51 Hatch Shell Concerts 115
52 Hemlock Gorge Reservation 117
53 Honan-Allston Branch Library 119
54 Houghton Garden 121
55 Howard Ulfelder, MD, Healing Garden 123
56 Hungry I 125

57 Inn at Castle Hill on the Crane Estate 126
58 The Institute of Contemporary Art, Boston 129
59 Isabella Stewart Gardner Museum 131

60 Jamaica Pond 134
61 John F. Kennedy Memorial Park 136
62 John Joseph Moakley U.S. Courthouse 138
63 Jordan Hall, New England Conservatory 141
64 Judson B. Coit Observatory, Boston University 143

65 Kaji Aso Studio Institute for the Arts 145
66 Kelleher Rose Garden 147
67 Kevin W. Fitzgerald Park 149

68 Lala Rokh 151
69 Lannan Ship Model Gallery 152
70 Lechmere Canal Park 154
71 Lewis Wharf Hidden Garden 156
72 Longfellow House Gardens 158
73 Lyman Estate Greenhouses 160

74 Massachusetts Avenue Bridge Moonrise 162
75 Massachusetts College of Art and Design Galleries 164

76 Massachusetts Institute of Technology Chapel 166
77 McCormick Gallery, Boston Architectural College 168
78 Millennium Park 170
79 Monastery of the Society of Saint John the Evangelist 172
80 Mothers' Walk, Rose F. Kennedy Greenway 174
81 Mount Auburn Cemetery 176
82 Mount Auburn Cemetery, Washington Tower 178
83 Mount Auburn Street, Middle Eastern Markets 180
84 Museum of Fine Arts, Boston 182

85 New England Aquarium, Harbor Seals 184
86 New England Wildflower Society, Garden in the Woods 186
87 Norman B. Leventhal Park 188
88 North End Shopping 190
89 North Point Park 192

90 Oceanic House, Star Island 194
91 Old South Church, Chorus pro Musica Sing 196
92 154 Lounge, Back Bay Hotel 198
93 101 Merrimac Street Atrium 200

94 Panopticon Gallery 202
95 Paul Revere Mall 204
96 Peter Faneuil House Garden 206
97 Piers Park 208
98 Portsmouth Excursion 210
99 Provincetown Excursion 213
100 Prudential Center South Garden 216

101 Radcliffe Institute for Advanced Study, Sunken Garden 218
102 Raven Used Books 220
103 Restaurant Dante 222
104 Ricky's Flower Market 224

105 Riverway 226
106 Rose Art Museum 228

107 Sacred Space, Northeastern University 230
108 Seaport Parks 232
109 Southwest Corridor Park 235
110 SoWa District 237
111 Swan Boats of Boston 239

112 Tavern at Granite Links Golf Club at Quarry Hills 241
113 Tower Hill Botanic Garden 243
114 Trident Booksellers & Café 246
115 Trinity Church Boston, Organ Concerts 248
116 Trinity Church Boston, St. Francis Garden 250

117 UpStairs on the Square 252
118 Uptown Espresso Caffe 254

119 Vilna Shul 256

120 Wellesley College Botanic Gardens 258
121 World's End 260

dedication

For my dear family and friends,
whose love and support make my heart a peaceful place.

acknowledgments

$\mathcal{C}$ ountless people—past and present, famous and unknown, individuals and organizations—have contributed and continue to offer the vision, passion, and tireless efforts to create, preserve, and maintain the special places that abound in Boston and in our corner of New England. They come from many avenues of life: public servants and private philanthropists, architects and landscape designers, university presidents and museum directors, artists and advocates for the arts. Together they are stewards for natural places, historic preservation, and open space and public access. Alongside them are myriad staff and volunteers who protect and care for these treasures.

To you all, I owe my deepest gratitude.

Additionally, so many friends and acquaintances were generous with their time—providing suggestions and advice and even accompanying me on my journeys to the places described in this book. Special thanks go to Blue Magruder, Jon and Jessie Panek, Elliot and Jeri Goldberg, Jeri Quinzio, and Christopher J. Hawes.

I also want to thank Phoebe Morad for introducing me to the amazing Al Maze, Boston tour guide and raconteur extraordinaire. He not only shared his vast knowledge of the city but also acted as my personal escort to his beloved Forest Hills Cemetery, among other places. Kudos to you, too, Al.

There are many people I met in the course of my research who earned my appreciation by returning phone calls, responding to e-mails, and offering helpful information and guidance. Among them are Robert Tullis, Patrice Tidesco, Kate Finnegan, and others too numerous to mention. But they include innkeepers, museum docents, park rangers, and fellow seekers of serenity.

I also want to thank my clients and coworkers who provided enthusiasm and support, even when my research took me away from the office.

To my editor, dear friend, and college sorority "mom," Susan Haynes, this book would not have been possible without your encouragement, patience, and amazing professional skills.

Finally, to Robin Schweikart and Dave Farrington, my sister and brother-in-law: Thank you for your generosity and unconditional support in this and all my endeavors, as well as for your wisdom, sense of humor, and boundless love. I am forever grateful.

introduction

There was once a king who offered a prize to the artist who could paint the best picture of peace. Many artists tried. The king looked at all of the pictures. After much deliberation he was down to the last two. He had to choose between them.

One picture was of a calm lake. The lake was a perfect mirror for the peaceful mountains that towered around it. Overhead, fluffy white clouds floated in a blue sky. Everyone who saw this picture said that it was the perfect picture of peace.

The second picture had mountains too. These mountains were rugged and bare. Above was an angry gray sky from which rain fell. Lightning flashed. Down the side of the mountain tumbled a foaming waterfall. This did not appear to be a peaceful place at all. But, when the king looked closely, he saw that behind the waterfall was a tiny bush growing in the rock. Inside the bush, a mother bird had built her nest. There, in the midst of the rush of angry water, sat the mother bird on her nest. She was the perfect picture of peace.

The king chose the second picture. "Because," he explained, "peace is not only in a place where there is no noise, trouble, or hard work. Peace is in the midst of things as they are, when there is calm in your heart. That is the real meaning of peace."

—This version of the traditional tale "Portrait of Peace" is shared courtesy of storyteller Linda Spitzer (**storyqueen.com**)

For too many of us, life today is like the second picture described in the wise old tale above. There are pressures of work and too many obligations. Anger and mean-spiritedness have engulfed our public discourse. We are beset by noise and trouble. More than ever, we need ways to find peace "in the midst of things as they are," places where we can find the calm in our hearts that refreshes our spirit, restores our balance, and renews our ability to appreciate the joys and meet the challenges of daily life.

This book describes 121 of what I've come to think of as my birds on the nest. Some sites likely will be familiar to you; others, unknown; still others, I hope, will offer new ways for you to experience Boston's most beloved traditions. A surprising number are in urban areas—just a brief walk, ride, or drive from the places many of us work or live. Throughout the Boston area, you can immerse yourself in a tranquil landscape; lose yourself in art or music; or take a quiet stroll, even if only for a quick break.

For those who have a few hours, a day, or even a weekend, there are blissful spots both in and out of the city where you can picnic, paddle, bike, go wandering, or relax—whatever suits your fancy. How blessed we are to live in a locale where there are so many tempting places to savor—and so many different types of peacefulness.

In the course of my explorations, I discovered too many special places for one book. If you're disappointed that your favorites are not listed here, and you're willing to share, I'll post them on the Peaceful Places Boston blog (**peacefulplacesboston.blogspot.com**) and the Peaceful Places Boston Facebook page.

I can't define peacefulness. But to paraphrase the old adage, I know it when I feel it. Sometimes, a total calm settles over me. Other times, there's an element of exhilaration. Always, there's a heartfelt gratitude—for the place, for being there, and for being mindfully aware: a whisper of thanks to the universe.

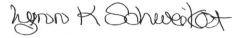

P.S. I have included public transportation options in the "essentials" sections for entries throughout this book. If travel by bus, train, subway, or ferry is not available to a particular site, or if multiple transfers would undermine the tranquil experience, you will see "n/a" (not applicable). Otherwise, you typically will see "T," local vernacular for the Massachusetts Bay Transit Authority (MBTA). Where pertinent, some entries note travel options available from other companies. (See page xvii for more about public transportation.)

three paths to 121 peaceful places

*I*n *Peaceful Places: Boston,* author Lynn Schweikart serves up 121 locales for a few hours of quiet time in the greater metro area and farther afield. To make it easy for you to find an entry that suits your mood and desired neighborhood or type of place, we have organized the sites in three different ways.

the path BY CATEGORY

The Peaceful Places by Category guide (see page xviii) organizes the sites into 12 different groups, as listed below. The full text for each destination also includes its category at the top of that individual entry. In many cases it was difficult to classify a place, as it might be a historic site in an outdoor habitat with a scenic vista that feels like a spiritual enclave that is an urban surprise where you can take an enchanting walk! But we tagged each of the sites as seemed most fitting for the focus of the author's description.

Day Trips & Overnights	Outdoor Habitats	Scenic Vistas
Enchanting Walks	Parks & Gardens	Shops & Services
Historic Sites	Quiet Tables	Spiritual Enclaves
Museums & Galleries	Reading Rooms	Urban Surprises

the path BY AREA

The Peaceful Places by Area guide (see page xxiii) and maps (pages xxviii–xxxix) locate sites according to 12 geographic divisions and their immediate environs:

Back Bay (MAP ONE)

Beacon Hill (MAP TWO)

Downtown, North End, & Waterfront (MAP THREE)

Seaport, South Boston, South End, & Boston Harbor (MAP FOUR)

Fenway & Kenmore Square (MAP FIVE)

Allston, Cambridge, & Watertown (MAP SIX)

East Cambridge, Somerville, Charlestown, & East Boston (MAP SEVEN)

Jamaica Plain, West Roxbury, Newton, & Brookline (MAP EIGHT)

West of Boston (MAP NINE)

North of Boston (MAP TEN)

South of Boston (MAP ELEVEN)

Farther Afield (MAP TWELVE)

the path ALPHANUMERICALLY

Beginning on page 1, each entry unfolds in the main text in alphabetical order and is numbered in sequence. The number travels with that entry throughout the book in the table of contents (see page v), in the Peaceful Places by Category guide (see page xviii), in the Peaceful Places by Area guide (see page xxiii), and on the maps (see pages xxviii–xxxix).

PEACEFULNESS RATINGS

Preceding the main text for each profile, listed information notes the entry's area, map number, and category. This capsule information also includes the author's rating for the site, on a scale of one to three stars, as follows:

✪ ✪ ✪   Heavenly anytime

✪ ✪   Almost always sublime

✪   Tranquil if visited as described in the entry—during times of day, week, season, and so on—and possibly avoided at certain times

ESSENTIALS

At the end of each entry, you will find the destination's full address; telephone number; website address; cost of entry or a range of prices for menu items or other expenses; hours; and public transportation choices. Hours and fees or prices are commonly subject to change, so call to verify before visiting a site.

Regarding public transportation: As the author points out in the postscript in her introduction, on page xiv, "n/a" (not applicable) denotes destinations not reachable—or not easily accessible—via these services. And as all Bostonians and other urban dwellers know, public transportation schedules and routes are subject to change. The routes and connections provided are up-to-date at press time, but please check the appropriate websites to be sure that you have the latest information for your own journeys.

The subway, bus, commuter rail, and ferry lines operated by the Massachusetts Bay Transit Authority provide service to more than 175 cities and towns in Eastern Massachusetts. For more information on the diverse public transportation systems and trip planning in Boston and vicinity, visit **mbta.com.** For destinations in this book that are served by other public transportation operators, visit the pertinent websites noted in the "essentials" sections for those *Peaceful Places* entries.

—The Publisher

peaceful places by category

DAY TRIPS & OVERNIGHTS

40 Fruitlands Museum (page 90)

44 Guest House at Field Farm (page 99)

57 Inn at Castle Hill on the Crane Estate (page 126)

90 Oceanic House, Star Island (page 194)

98 Portsmouth Excursion (page 210)

99 Provincetown Excursion (page 213)

113 Tower Hill Botanic Garden (page 243)

ENCHANTING WALKS

7   Beacon Hill Stroll (page 15)

12 Boston HarborWalk, Downtown to North End (page 27)

24 Commonwealth Avenue Mall (page 54)

29 deCordova Sculpture Park and Museum (page 65)

36 Forest Hills Cemetery (page 81)

81 Mount Auburn Cemetery (page 176)

109 Southwest Corridor Park (page 235)

HISTORIC SITES

9   Boston Athenæum (page 20)

23 Codman Estate (page 52)

30 Dorchester Heights (page 68)

32 Ether Dome, Massachusetts General Hospital (page 72)

33 Faneuil Hall (page 74)

73 Lyman Estate Greenhouses (page 160)

95 Paul Revere Mall (page 204)

MUSEUMS & GALLERIES

1   Addison Gallery of American Art (page 1)

45 Guild of Boston Artists (page 102)

49 Harvard Museum of Natural History and Peabody Museum of Archaeology and Ethnology (page 110)

58 The Institute of Contemporary Art, Boston (page 129)

59 Isabella Stewart Gardner Museum (page 131)

75 Massachusetts College of Art and Design Galleries (page 164)

77 McCormick Gallery, Boston Architectural College (page 168)

84 Museum of Fine Arts, Boston (page 182)

94 Panopticon Gallery (page 202)

106 Rose Art Museum (page 228)

OUTDOOR HABITATS

8 Belle Isle Marsh Reservation (page 18)

10 Boston Common, Frog Pond Skating (page 23)

11 Boston Harbor Islands National Park (page 25)

14 Boston Nature Center and Wildlife Sanctuary (page 32)

25 Condor Street Urban Wild (page 57)

28 D. Blakely Hoar Sanctuary (page 63)

43 Gropius House (page 97)

46 Habitat Education Center and Wildlife Sanctuary (page 104)

47 Hall's Pond Sanctuary and Amory Woods (page 106)

52 Hemlock Gorge Reservation (page 117)

60 Jamaica Pond (page 134)

78 Millennium Park (page 170)

86 New England Wildflower Society, Garden in the Woods (page 186)

121 World's End (page 260)

PARKS & GARDENS

4 Arnold Arboretum of Harvard University (page 8)

20 Chinatown Park (page 46)

22 City Square Park (page 50)

35 Fenway Victory Gardens (page 79)

38 Franklin Square (page 86)

54 Houghton Garden (page 121)

PARKS & GARDENS *(continued)*

61   John F. Kennedy Memorial Park (page 136)

66   Kelleher Rose Garden (page 147)

70   Lechmere Canal Park (page 154)

72   Longfellow House Gardens (page 158)

87   Norman B. Leventhal Park (page 188)

89   North Point Park (page 192)

101   Radcliffe Institute for Advanced Study, Sunken Garden (page 218)

105   Riverway (page 226)

108   Seaport Parks (page 232)

111   Swan Boats of Boston (page 239)

120   Wellesley College Botanic Gardens (page 258)

QUIET TABLES

5   B&G Oysters (page 11)

26   Copley Plaza Hotel Oak Room (page 59)

31   L'Espalier Salon (page 70)

56   Hungry I (page 125)

68   Lala Rokh (page 151)

92   154 Lounge, Back Bay Hotel (page 198)

103   Restaurant Dante (page 222)

112   Tavern at Granite Links Golf Club at Quarry Hills (page 241)

117   UpStairs on the Square (page 252)

118   Uptown Espresso Caffe (page 254)

READING ROOMS

6   Bates Hall, Boston Public Library (page 13)

13   Boston Marine Society and Shipyard Park (page 30)

39   French Cultural Center of Boston (page 88)

53   Honan-Allston Branch Library (page 119)

SCENIC VISTAS

19   Charles River Kayaking (page 43)

21   Christian Science Center Reflecting Pool (page 48)

37   470 Atlantic Avenue Observation Deck (page 84)

41   Gloucester Street Dock (page 93)

55   Howard Ulfelder, MD, Healing Garden (page 123)

67   Kevin W. Fitzgerald Park (page 149)

74   Massachusetts Avenue Bridge Moonrise (page 162)

82   Mount Auburn Cemetery, Washington Tower (page 178)

97   Piers Park (page 208)

SHOPS & SERVICES

2   Allandale Farm and Roadside Stand (page 4)

27   Copley Square Farmers' Market (page 61)

50   Harvard Square Bookstores (page 112)

69   Lannan Ship Model Gallery (page 152)

83   Mount Auburn Street, Middle Eastern Markets (page 180)

88   North End Shopping (page 190)

102 Raven Used Books (page 220)

104 Ricky's Flower Market (page 224)

110 SoWa District (page 237)

114 Trident Booksellers & Café (page 246)

SPIRITUAL ENCLAVES

3   Arlington Street Church (page 6)

42   Greater Boston Buddhist Cultural Center (page 95)

48   Harvard Divinity School Quadrangle Labyrinth (page 108)

65   Kaji Aso Studio Institute for the Arts (page 145)

76   Massachusetts Institute of Technology Chapel (page 166)

79   Monastery of the Society of Saint John the Evangelist (page 172)

SPIRITUAL ENCLAVES *(continued)*

107   Sacred Space, Northeastern University (page 230)

115   Trinity Church Boston, Organ Concerts (page 248)

119   Vilna Shul (page 256)

URBAN SURPRISES

15   Boston Public Library Courtyard (page 34)

16   Cafe 939, Berklee School of Music (page 36)

17   Cambridge Center Garage Roof Garden (page 38)

18   Charles River Gondola Ride (page 40)

34   Fenway Park (page 76)

51   Hatch Shell Concerts (page 115)

62   John Joseph Moakley U.S. Courthouse (page 138)

63   Jordan Hall, New England Conservatory (page 141)

64   Judson B. Coit Observatory, Boston University (page 143)

71   Lewis Wharf Hidden Garden (page 156)

80   Mothers' Walk, Rose F. Kennedy Greenway (page 174)

85   New England Aquarium, Harbor Seals (page 184)

91   Old South Church, Chorus pro Musica Sing (page 196)

93   101 Merrimac Street Atrium (page 200)

96   Peter Faneuil House Garden (page 206)

100   Prudential Center South Garden (page 216)

116   Trinity Church Boston, St. Francis Garden (page 250)

peaceful places by area

BACK BAY (Map One)

3	Arlington Street Church (page 6)
6	Bates Hall, Boston Public Library (page 13)
15	Boston Public Library Courtyard (page 34)
16	Cafe 939, Berklee School of Music (page 36)
18	Charles River Gondola Ride (page 40)
21	Christian Science Center Reflecting Pool (page 48)
24	Commonwealth Avenue Mall (see 24A and 24B) (page 54)
26	Copley Plaza Hotel Oak Room (page 59)
27	Copley Square Farmers' Market (page 61)
31	L'Espalier Salon (page 70)
39	French Cultural Center of Boston (page 88)
41	Gloucester Street Dock (page 93)
45	Guild of Boston Artists (page 102)
51	Hatch Shell Concerts (page 115)
77	McCormick Gallery, Boston Architectural College (page 168)
91	Old South Church, Chorus pro Musica Sing (page 196)
92	154 Lounge, Back Bay Hotel (page 198)
100	Prudential Center South Garden (page 216)
102	Raven Used Books (page 220)
111	Swan Boats of Boston (page 239)
114	Trident Booksellers & Café (page 246)
115	Trinity Church Boston, Organ Concerts (page 248)
116	Trinity Church Boston, St. Francis Garden (page 250)

BEACON HILL (Map Two)

7	Beacon Hill Stroll (page 15)
9	Boston Athenæum (page 20)
10	Boston Common, Frog Pond Skating (page 23)
32	Ether Dome, Massachusetts General Hospital (page 72)
55	Howard Ulfelder, MD, Healing Garden (page 123)

BEACON HILL (Map Two) *(continued)*

56   Hungry I (page 125)

68   Lala Rokh (page 151)

93   101 Merrimac Street Atrium (page 200)

96   Peter Faneuil House Garden (page 206)

119   Vilna Shul (page 256)

DOWNTOWN, NORTH END, & WATERFRONT (Map Three)

12   Boston HarborWalk, Downtown to North End (page 27)

20   Chinatown Park (page 46)

33   Faneuil Hall (page 74)

37   470 Atlantic Avenue Observation Deck (page 84)

69   Lannan Ship Model Gallery (page 152)

71   Lewis Wharf Hidden Garden (page 156)

80   Mothers' Walk, Rose F. Kennedy Greenway (page 174)

85   New England Aquarium, Harbor Seals (page 184)

87   Norman B. Leventhal Park (page 188)

88   North End Shopping (page 190)

95   Paul Revere Mall (page 204)

SEAPORT, SOUTH BOSTON, SOUTH END, & BOSTON HARBOR (Map Four)

5   B&G Oysters (page 11)

11   Boston Harbor Islands National Park (page 25)

30   Dorchester Heights (page 68)

38   Franklin Square (page 86)

58   The Institute of Contemporary Art, Boston (page 129)

62   John Joseph Moakley U.S. Courthouse (page 138)

108   Seaport Parks (page 232)

109   Southwest Corridor Park (page 235)

110   SoWa District (page 237)

118   Uptown Espresso Caffe (page 254)

FENWAY & KENMORE SQUARE (Map Five)

34   Fenway Park (page 76)

35   Fenway Victory Gardens (page 79)

53   Honan-Allston Branch Library (also see Map Six) (page 119)

59   Isabella Stewart Gardner Museum (page 131)

63   Jordan Hall, New England Conservatory (page 141)

64   Judson B. Coit Observatory, Boston University (page 143)

65   Kaji Aso Studio Institute for the Arts (page 145)

66   Kelleher Rose Garden (page 147)

84   Museum of Fine Arts, Boston (page 182)

94   Panopticon Gallery (page 202)

105   Riverway (also see 105A and 105B on Map Eight) (page 226)

107   Sacred Space, Northeastern University (page 230)

ALLSTON, CAMBRIDGE, & WATERTOWN (Map Six)

42   Greater Boston Buddhist Cultural Center (page 95)

48   Harvard Divinity School Quadrangle Labyrinth (page 108)

49   Harvard Museum of Natural History and Peabody Museum of Archaeology and Ethnology (page 110)

50   Harvard Square Bookstores (page 112)

53   Honan-Allston Branch Library (also see Map Five) (page 119)

61   John F. Kennedy Memorial Park (page 136)

72   Longfellow House Gardens (page 158)

74   Massachusetts Avenue Bridge Moonrise (page 162)

76   Massachusetts Institute of Technology Chapel (page 166)

79   Monastery of the Society of Saint John the Evangelist (page 172)

81   Mount Auburn Cemetery (page 176)

82   Mount Auburn Cemetery, Washington Tower (page 178)

83   Mount Auburn Street, Middle Eastern Markets (page 180)

101   Radcliffe Institute for Advanced Study, Sunken Garden (page 218)

117   UpStairs on the Square (page 252)

EAST CAMBRIDGE, SOMERVILLE, CHARLESTOWN, & EAST BOSTON (Map Seven)

   8   Belle Isle Marsh Reservation (page 18)
  13   Boston Marine Society and Shipyard Park (page 30)
  17   Cambridge Center Garage Roof Garden (page 38)
  19   Charles River Kayaking (see 19A on this map; also see 19B on Map Eight) (page 43)
  22   City Square Park (page 50)
  25   Condor Street Urban Wild (page 57)
  70   Lechmere Canal Park (page 154)
  89   North Point Park (page 192)
  97   Piers Park (page 208)
 103   Restaurant Dante (page 222)
 104   Ricky's Flower Market (page 224)

JAMAICA PLAIN, WEST ROXBURY, NEWTON, & BROOKLINE (Map Eight)

   2   Allandale Farm and Roadside Stand (page 4)
   4   Arnold Arboretum of Harvard University (page 8)
  14   Boston Nature Center and Wildlife Sanctuary (page 32)
  19   Charles River Kayaking (see 19B on this map; also see 19A on Map Seven) (page 43)
  28   D. Blakely Hoar Sanctuary (page 63)
  36   Forest Hills Cemetery (page 81)
  47   Hall's Pond Sanctuary and Amory Woods (page 106)
  52   Hemlock Gorge Reservation (page 117)
  54   Houghton Garden (page 121)
  60   Jamaica Pond (page 134)
  67   Kevin W. Fitzgerald Park (page 149)
  75   Massachusetts College of Art and Design Galleries (page 164)
  78   Millennium Park (page 170)
 105   Riverway (see 105A and 105B on this map; also see 105 on Map Five) (page 226)

WEST OF BOSTON (Map Nine)

23   Codman Estate (page 52)

29   deCordova Sculpture Park and Museum (page 65)

43   Gropius House (page 97)

46   Habitat Education Center and Wildlife Sanctuary (page 104)

73   Lyman Estate Greenhouses (page 160)

86   New England Wildflower Society, Garden in the Woods (page 186)

106   Rose Art Museum (page 228)

120   Wellesley College Botanic Gardens (page 258)

NORTH OF BOSTON (Map Ten)

1   Addison Gallery of American Art (page 1)

57   Inn at Castle Hill on the Crane Estate (page 126)

90   Oceanic House, Star Island (page 194)

98   Portsmouth Excursion (page 210)

SOUTH OF BOSTON (Map Eleven)

99   Provincetown Excursion (page 213)

112   Tavern at Granite Links Golf Club at Quarry Hills (page 241)

121   World's End (page 260)

FARTHER AFIELD (Map Twelve)

40   Fruitlands Museum (page 90)

44   Guest House at Field Farm (page 99)

113   Tower Hill Botanic Garden (page 243)

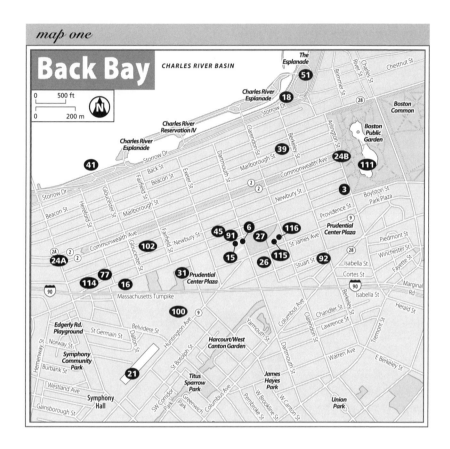

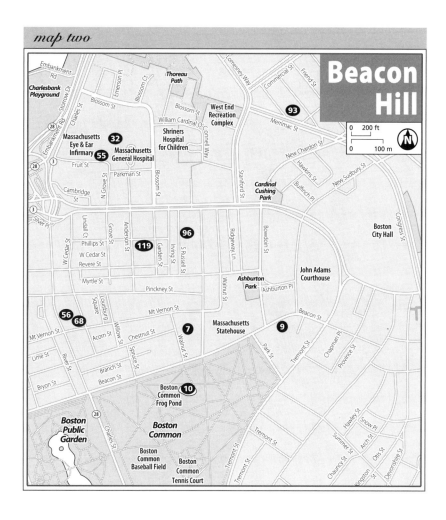

map two

Beacon Hill

0   200 ft
0   100 m

Embankment Rd
Charlesbank Playground
Storrow Dr
Emerson Pl
Blossom Ct
Thoreau Path
Lomesney Way
Commercial St
Friend St
Charles St
Blossom St
Blossom St
West End Recreation Complex
93
Merrimac St
William Cardinal O'Connell Way
28
Massachusetts Eye & Ear Infirmary   32
Shriners Hospital for Children
New Chardon St
Embankment Rd
Massachusetts General Hospital   55
Hawkins St
3
Fruit St
Blossom St
Bulfinch Pl
New Sudbury St
28
Parkman St
Stamford St
Cardinal Cushing Park
Cambridge St
N Grove St
Boston City Hall
3
Silver Pl
Lindall Ct
Grove St
Anderson St
96
Ridgeway Ln
Bowdoin St
Congress St
W Cedar St
Phillips St
119
Garden St
Irving St
S Russell St
W Cedar St
Revere St
John Adams Courthouse
Myrtle St
Ashburton Park
Walnut St
Pinckney St
Ashburton Pl
Louisburg Square
Mt Vernon St
Beacon St
56   68
Willow St
7
Massachusetts Statehouse
9
Mt Vernon St
Acorn St
Chestnut St
Walnut St
Chapman Pl
Province St
Lime St
River St
Spruce St
Park St
Tremont St
Branch St
Beacon St
Bryon St
Boston Common Frog Pond   10
Hawley St
Snow Pl
Boston Public Garden
28
Charles St
Boston Common
Tremont St
Summer St
Arch St
Otis St
Boston Common Baseball Field
Boston Common Tennis Court
Tremont St
Tremont St
Chauncy St
Kingston St
Devonshire St

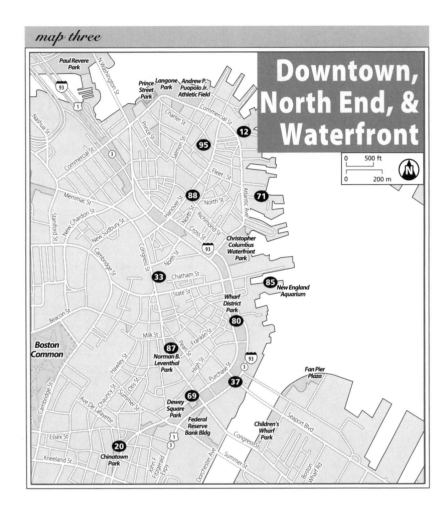

map three

Downtown, North End, & Waterfront

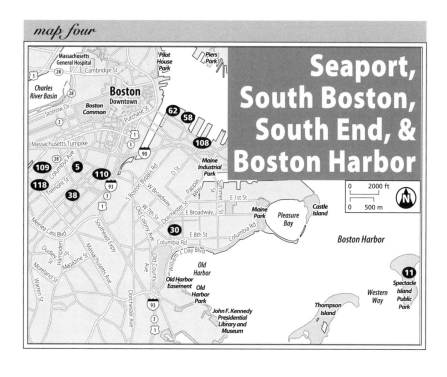

map four

Seaport, South Boston, South End, & Boston Harbor

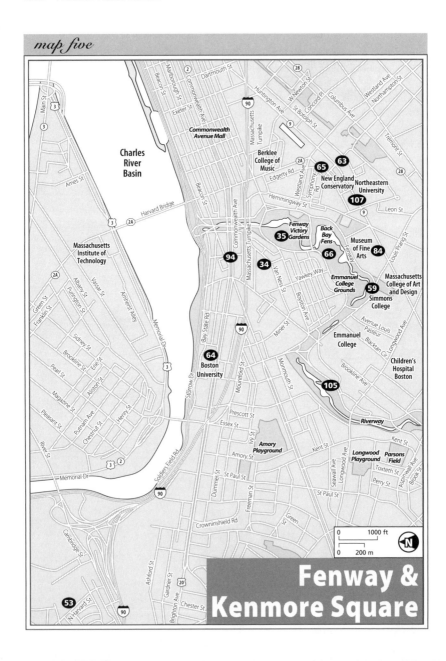

map five

Charles
River
Basin

Commonwealth
Avenue Mall

Massachusetts
Institute of
Technology

Berklee
College of
Music

65 **63**
New England **107** Northeastern
Conservatory **107** University

Fenway
Victory
Gardens
35

Back
Bay
Fens
66

Museum
of Fine **84**
Arts

Massachusetts
College of Art
and Design
59
Simmons
College

Emmanuel
College
Grounds

94

34

64
Boston
University

Emmanuel
College

Children's
Hospital
Boston

105

Riverway

Amory
Playground

Longwood
Playground   Parsons
Field

0   1000 ft
0   200 m

53

Fenway &
Kenmore Square

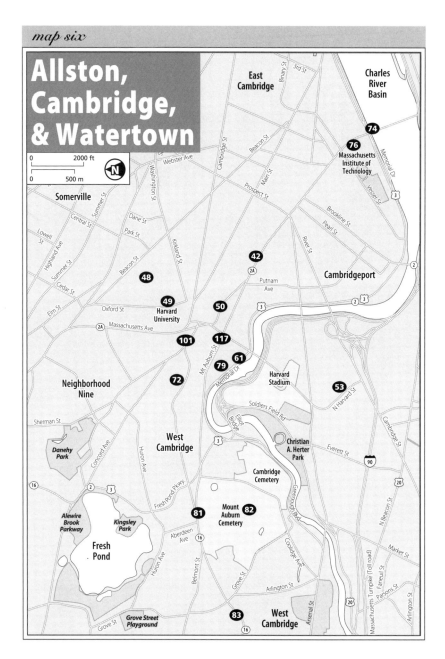

map six

Allston, Cambridge, & Watertown

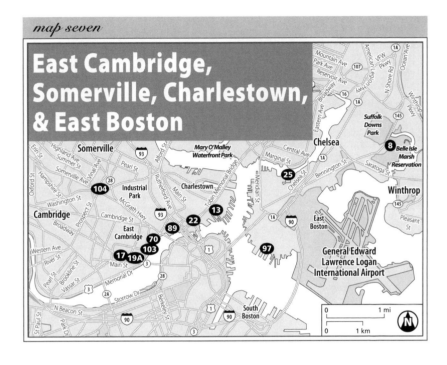

map seven

East Cambridge, Somerville, Charlestown, & East Boston

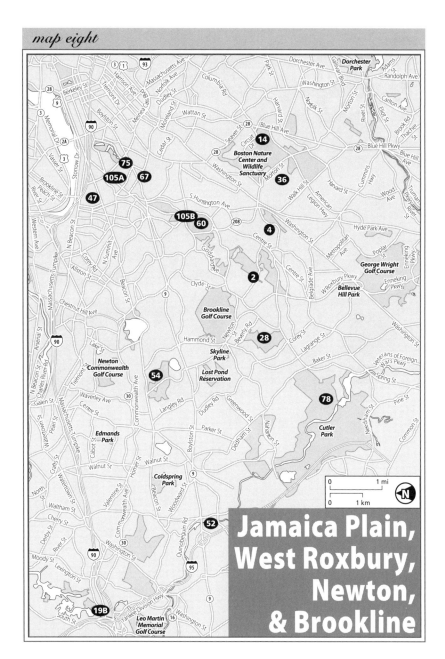

map eight

Jamaica Plain, West Roxbury, Newton, & Brookline

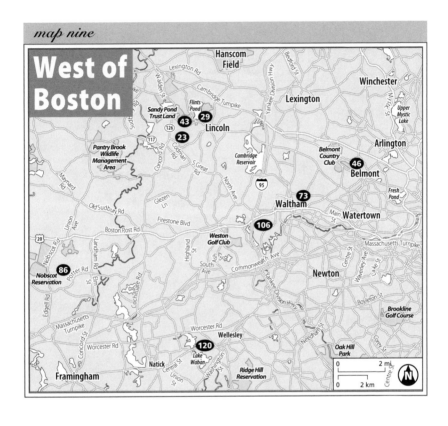

map nine

West of Boston

Hanscom Field

Winchester

Lexington Rd

Walders St

Cambridge Turnpike

Lexington

Bedford St

Mystic St

Upper Mystic Lake

Sandy Pond Trust Land

Flints Pond

29

43

126

Lincoln

117

Codman Rd

23

Pantry Brook Wildlife Management Area

Concord Rd

S Great Rd

Cambridge Reservoir

Belmont Country Club

46

Arlington

Belmont

North Ave

95

Fresh Pond

Glezen Ln

Maynard Rd

Old Sudbury Rd

Union Ave

Firestone Blvd

73

Waltham

Main St

Watertown

106

Boston Post Rd

20

Nobscot Rd

Landham Rd

Weston Golf Club

Highland St

Massachusetts Turnpike

Centre St

Waverley St

Lake St

Elm

86

Nobscot Reservation

Potter Rd

South Ave

Commonwealth Ave

Yankee Division Hwy

Newton

Boylston St

Brookline Golf Course

Edgell Rd

Cochituate Rd

Massachusetts Turnpike

Concord St

Worcester Rd

Worcester Rd

Wellesley

120

Lake Waban

Natick

Central St

Union St

Washington St

Needham St

Corey St

Ridge Hill Reservation

Oak Hill Park

Framingham

0   2 mi.

0   2 km

Centre St

Centre St

N

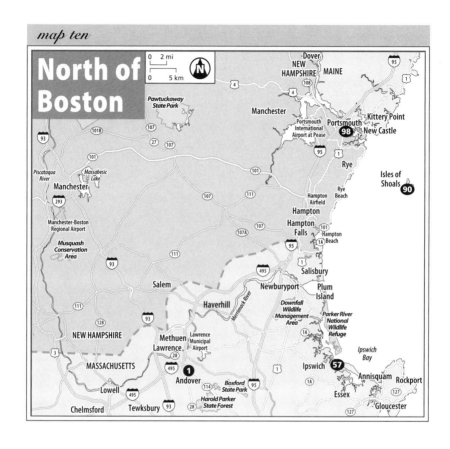

map ten

North of Boston

0 2 mi
0 5 km

Pawtuckaway State Park

Dover
NEW
HAMPSHIRE MAINE

95

1

108

Manchester

4

4

Portsmouth
International
Airport at Pease

Portsmouth Kittery Point

98 New Castle

101B

107

93

27 107

95

101

Rye

Piscataqua
River

Massabesic
Lake

101

Isles of
Shoals 90

Manchester

107

111

Rye
Beach

Hampton
Airfield

293

107

Manchester-Boston
Regional Airport

Hampton

**Musquash
Conservation
Area**

111

107A

Hampton
Falls 101

Hampton
Beach

1A

93

95

Salem

495

1 Salisbury

111

Haverhill

Merrimack River

Newburyport Plum
Island

*Downfall
Wildlife
Management
Area*

Parker River
National
Wildlife
Refuge

128

1A

111

93

NEW HAMPSHIRE

3

Methuen Lawrence
Municipal
Airport

Ipswich
Bay

Lawrence

28

Ipswich 57

MASSACHUSETTS

1

Annisquam Rockport

495

1

1A

Lowell

Andover 114

Boxford
State Park

95

Essex Gloucester

495

28

Harold Parker
State Forest

Chelmsford Tewksbury 93

127

map eleven

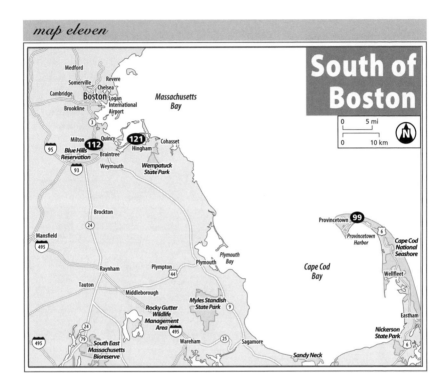

map twelve

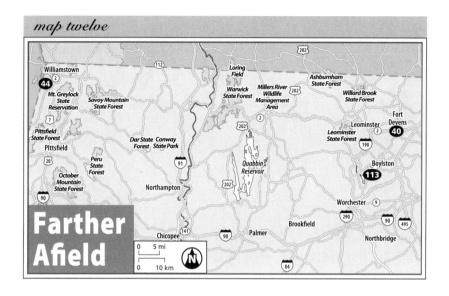

Williamstown
44
Mt. Greylock State Reservation
Savoy Mountain State Forest
Pittsfield State Forest
Pittsfield
Peru State Forest
October Mountain State Forest
90
20
Dar State Forest
Conway State Park
Northampton
91
112
Loring Field
Warwick State Forest
Millers River Wildlife Management Area
202
202
Quabbin Reservoir
202
202
Ashburnham State Forest
Willard Brook State Forest
Leominster
Leominster State Forest
190
Fort Devens
40
Boylston
113
Worcester
9
290
90
495
Brookfield
Northbridge
Chicopee
141
90
Palmer
84

Farther Afield

0   5 mi
0   10 km
N

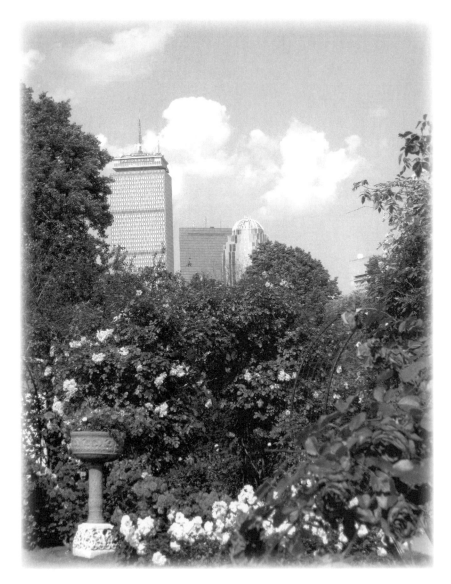

Kelleher Rose Garden (see page 147)

peaceful places
Boston

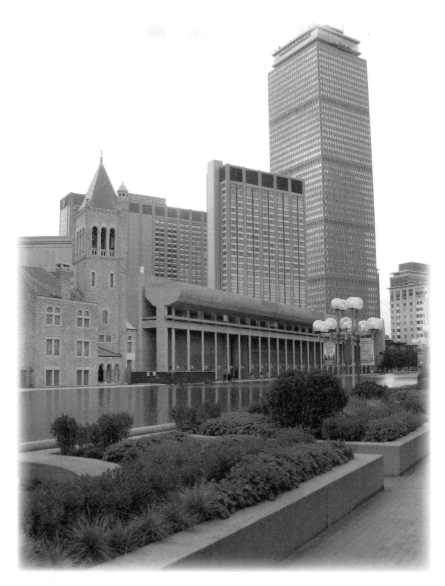

Christian Science Center Reflecting Pool (see page 48)

peaceful place 1

ADDISON GALLERY OF AMERICAN ART

Phillips Academy, Andover, MA (MAP TEN)

CATEGORY ⌣ museums & galleries ✪ ✪ ✪

To find what many consider the world's finest permanent collection of American art, just venture north of Boston to the Addison Gallery of American Art, on the leafy campus of Phillips Academy. Don't let the name *gallery* fool you. This is actually a rare gem of a *museum*, possessing nearly 17,000 paintings, photographs, sculptures, and other works of American art from the 18th century onward.

The collection is too large to be exhibited in its entirety; however, at any given time, there are enough varied treasures on display in the intimate gallery spaces to delight even the most jaded art lover. On one visit, I saw three Winslow Homers, a Georgia O'Keeffe, and works by Jackson Pollock, John Singer Sargent, and Ansel Adams, among many others. And that was just in one room!

Because it has a somewhat lower profile than other art institutions in the area, the Addison is rarely crowded, even on weekends. It's not unusual to find yourself alone in a gallery, with plenty of opportunity to take your time and slowly absorb the experience. One of the enhancements is that, despite its stature, the museum is decidedly unstuffy. If the sofas and easy chairs that are usually placed throughout the galleries add a homey touch, it's because they literally came from the living room of an early benefactress.

Want to know more about the art you're seeing? Thanks to the Addison's educational focus, the library overflows with books on the artists whose work appears in the collection. Select a volume and settle into a comfortable chair in the light-filled Museum Learning Center, which is usually so quiet that it has become a favorite study spot for Phillips Academy students. Also take some time to check out the Addison's green roof and admire the 10 blown-glass spheres by Seattle-based artist Dale Chihuly.

If all that art makes you yearn for a little refreshment, the historic Andover Inn is just a brief walk away on Chapel Avenue. Or perhaps you'd prefer to escape into a real landscape? The Trustees of Reservations' Charles W. Ward property—with its hiking trails, solstice stones, quaking bog, and views toward Boston—is less than 2 miles away.

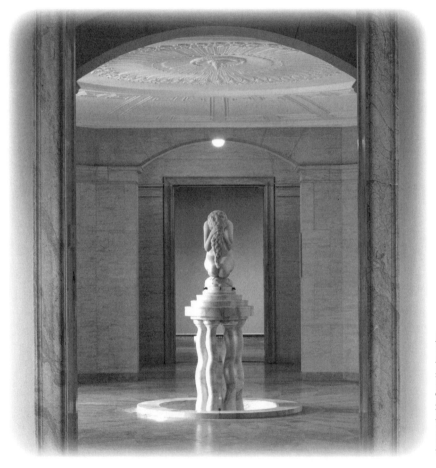

The marble Venus Anadyomene *by Paul Manship at The Addison Gallery of American Art*

essentials

Phillips Academy, 180 Main Street, Andover, MA 01810

(978) 749-4015

addisongallery.org

$ Free

Tuesday–Saturday, 10 a.m.–5 p.m.; Sunday, 1–5 p.m.; closed national holidays, the month of August, and December 24

n/a

peaceful place 2

ALLANDALE FARM AND ROADSIDE STAND

Jamaica Plain, Boston/Brookline, MA (MAP EIGHT)

CATEGORY ⌣ shops & services ✪

*J*ust off busy Centre Street, near the Veterans of Foreign Wars Parkway, you'll find Allandale Farm. Not only is it the city's last working farm, but it has also been in operation continuously for seven generations. In addition to chickens and a small herd of Scottish Highland cattle, nearly 30 acres of vegetables—including potatoes, leeks, squash, pumpkins, and 30–40 varieties of heirloom tomatoes—thrive here.

Though the fields themselves are off-limits to visitors, Allandale operates a garden center and farm stand with the laid-back, friendly atmosphere of an old-fashioned

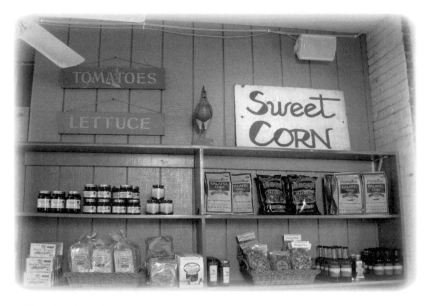

Victuals at the roadside farm stand

country store. Here, in addition to the farm's seasonal produce and eggs laid by free-range chickens, you can choose from a tempting selection of locally crafted artisanal foods and plantings. They include breads and baked goods, cheeses, coffee, and ice cream, as well as bedding plants, perennials, and herbs for your garden or window box. On Wednesday afternoons, you'll even find local seafood fresh off the truck from Jordan Bros. of Gloucester. The farm stand is also the perfect place to pick up the fixings for a truly authentic New England Thanksgiving. Just remember to order a fresh turkey from Allandale Farm well in advance.

Should you yearn to breathe in a little more of that refreshing country air, you're welcome to take a leisurely stroll around the nearby lily pond, as long as you respect the NO TRESPASSING signs beyond it.

essentials

259 Allandale Road, Brookline, MA 02467

(617) 524-1531

allandalefarm.com

$ Free

April–December 23: Monday–Friday, 10 a.m.–6:30 p.m.; Saturday–Sunday, 9 a.m.–6 p.m.

T: Bus 38 (Wren Street/Forest Hills Station) to the stop at corner of Centre Street and Allandale Road or Bus 51 (Cleveland Circle/Forest Hills Station) to the stop at corner of Grove Street and Allandale Road; then walk 0.5 mile down Allandale Road

peaceful place 3

ARLINGTON STREET CHURCH

Back Bay, Boston (MAP ONE)

CATEGORY ◡ spiritual enclaves ✪ ✪ ✪

*L*ong before little blue boxes and Holly Golightly, the name Tiffany was synonymous with exquisitely crafted stained glass. Other than congregation members, not many people are aware that the sanctuary of the Back Bay's Unitarian Universalist Arlington Street Church is home to what has been called the largest collection of Tiffany stained glass windows in any one house of worship. That it's possible for one to make a private pilgrimage to experience these windows is an even better-kept secret. But as long as there's no other activity scheduled, with proper notice, you're welcome to enter the sanctuary and stay for as long as you desire.

According to the church's website, the original sanctuary was built with clear glass windows. The first of 20 proposed Tiffany windows, each designed to tell a particular story, was installed in 1899. By 1929, 16 were in place. When the Great Depression hit, further work was temporarily put on hold. But before the last of the windows could be completed, the Tiffany factory went out of business due to the founder's death. That's why, to this day, four clear glass windows remain in the sanctuary.

If you are lucky, the sanctuary lights will remain unlit when you visit. I say that because I think that the windows are best seen with daylight alone. Depending on the weather, time of day, and position of the sun, some are more illuminated than others. I like to walk by each window first, starting with the darkest and moving toward the brightest, upstairs and down. When finished, I seek out a seat that allows me to take in as many windows as possible and watch the sun do its magic.

The church is a big space, with the kind of enclosed box pews that were once common in New England churches. While I don't consider myself to be a particularly religious person, there's something about this hushed semidarkness punctuated by streams of colored light that touches me on a deeply spiritual level.

⌣ essentials

📧 351 Boylston Street, Boston, MA 02116   📞 (617) 536-7050; call for appointment

🌐 ascboston.org   💲 Free   🕐 Monday–Friday, 9 a.m.–5 p.m.

🚍 **T:** Green Line, any train, to Arlington

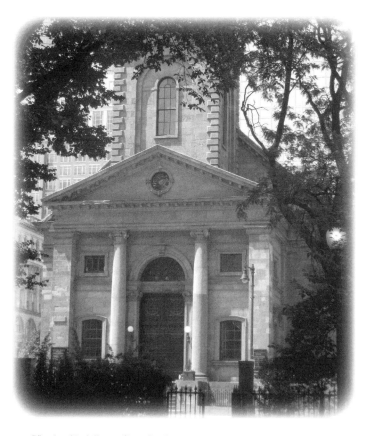

The church's Arlington Street facade

peaceful place 4

ARNOLD ARBORETUM OF HARVARD UNIVERSITY

Jamaica Plain, Boston (MAP EIGHT)

CATEGORY ↵ parks & gardens ✪

o many Bostonians, the Arnold Arboretum is best known for Lilac Sunday, which, like Red Sox Opening Day and Marathon Monday, has become something of an event of civic obligation. True, the sight and scent of nearly 400 lilacs simultaneously in bloom is something to behold. Yet the 265-acre arboretum, with nearly 15,000 individual plants arranged by botanical sequence, holds many charms. Peacefulness seekers can enjoy the flora without the crowds on most days other than Lilac Sunday.

To me, one of the most remarkable aspects of the arboretum is the way it combines scientific purpose with visual delight. While the plantings are grouped according to family, so you can easily compare one with another, the setting—with its varied terrain traversed by curving roads and pathways—inspires a profound connection to nature.

For instance, a walk through the linden collection, off the aptly named Linden Path, feels like entering a sacred grove. In July, the shade is deep and the fragrance, heavenly. Come late May, my spot of choice is Rhododendron Path. Nestled at the bottom of Hemlock Hill, it meanders along gurgling Bussey Brook, offering numerous places to pause and marvel at the bounty of blossoms and birdsong. In any season, I enjoy winding my way through Explorers Garden, off Bussey Hill. Here, you'll be surrounded by specimens raised from seeds collected in China and Japan in the early 1900s. Be sure to look for the Dove Tree on Chinese Path, which is especially breathtaking in May.

Of course, fall color here is spectacular. By all means, indulge in the temptation to climb the 240-foot Peters Hill and enjoy the panorama that stretches over Bussey Hill to downtown Boston. (But be warned: despite leash laws, it's a popular place for local pooches to run free.) The varied topography and vistas mean cross-country skiing and snowshoeing are wintertime delights throughout the arboretum, and the sight of snow-covered evergreens along Conifer Path is both magical and tranquil.

On weekends, when the main path by the visitor center bustles with activity, the best strategy for peacefulness is to head off to one of the more remote entryways, such as South Street Gate, Bussey Street Gate, or Poplar Gate. If you come by T, Washington Street Gate is just steps away.

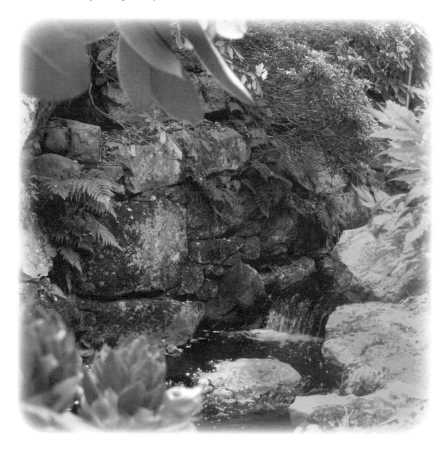

Bussey Brook in May

⌣ essentials

📧   125 Arborway, Boston, MA 02130

📞   (617) 524-1718

🌐   arboretum.harvard.edu

$ Free, though donations appreciated

🕐   **Grounds:** Daily, sunrise–sunset. **Visitor center:** Monday–Friday, 9 a.m.–4 p.m.;
      Saturday, 10 a.m.–4 p.m.; Sunday, noon–4 p.m.; closed holidays.

🚊   **T:** Orange Line to Forest Hills

peaceful place 5

B&G OYSTERS

South End, Boston (MAP FOUR)

CATEGORY ⌣ quiet tables ✪

&G Oysters is like a little seaside lobster shack that decided to grow up and move to the big city. Sure, there are still fried clams, calamari, and lobster on the menu, but with 12 or so different kinds of oysters and some Mediterranean-inspired appetizers and main dishes also on the list, the overall impression is classic and urbane, while still being friendly and easygoing. B&G is owned by executive chef Barbara Lynch,

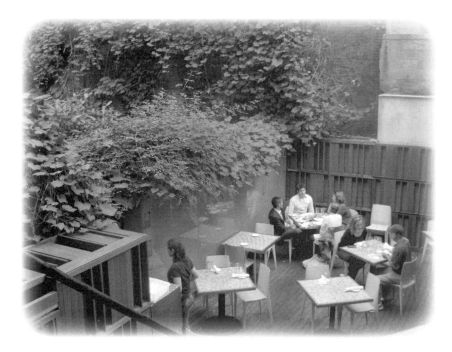

The patio during quiet times at B&G Oysters

the South Boston native who has transformed the local restaurant scene with inspired and eclectic offerings at her various restaurants.

Inside, B&G has the feel of an oyster bar in some nice but not touristy Parisian neighborhood. Though the dinner and bar scene can be a bit noisy, I've enjoyed many a quiet Saturday lunch here with friends from out of town. However, to me, B&G's truly special attraction is its outdoor patio. Tucked behind a stone wall off Waltham Street, it is open late April–October 31, depending on the weather. The ambience changes from dappled shade by day to candlelight by night. Grape- and trumpet vines twine up and over the walls. Even though you're only steps from the street, you feel sheltered from noise and traffic.

Because it's fun to share a couple dozen oysters, some roasted mussels, fried Ipswich clams, and lobster rolls, you'll likely want to come with friends. But the patio is also a place where you'd feel comfortable settling in with a book or your journal and dining alone.

Two warnings: The menu is pretty sparse if you're not a seafood lover. And the patio is small, with only eight tables, and no reservations are accepted for outside dining. Work around that by arriving for an early lunch or dinner, or unwind with some appetizers and a glass of wine in the late afternoon.

✌ essentials

✉	550 Tremont Street, Boston, MA 02116
✆	(617) 423-0550
⊕	bandgoysters.com
$	**Entrées:** $14–$27
⏱	Monday, 11:30 a.m.–10 p.m.; Tuesday–Friday, 11:30 a.m.–11 p.m.; Saturday, noon–11 p.m.; Sunday, noon–10 p.m.
🚆	**T:** Orange Line or Commuter Rail to Back Bay Station

peaceful place 6

BATES HALL, BOSTON PUBLIC LIBRARY

Back Bay, Boston (MAP ONE)

CATEGORY ↝ reading rooms ✪ ✪ ✪

*O*ne of Boston's most impressive interior spaces, the magnificent Bates Hall reading room spans 218 feet, nearly the entire length of the Dartmouth Street side of the library's main branch. With an ornate ceiling that soars to 50 feet, and 15 massive, arched windows, it's a bright spot on even the dreariest day.

Despite its size, Bates Hall is a surprisingly comfortable place. The green glass-shaded lamps on each of the 24 oak reading tables give off a cozy glow, especially after dark. Except when a tour group is passing through, the room has an atmosphere that's hushed

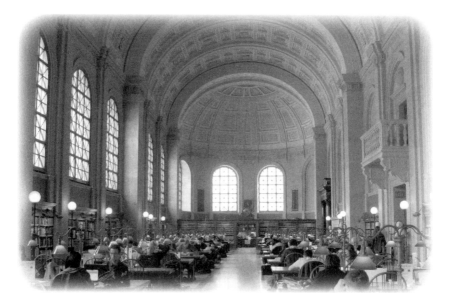

Savoring the silence at Bates Hall

but purposeful. You sense that you're in a place where important work is being accomplished, even if all you're doing is using the free Wi-Fi to chat with friends on Facebook.

Should you desire some solitary inspiration, I suggest visiting the luxuriously ornamental Abbey Room, where Edwin Austin Abbey's elaborate murals celebrate the quest for the Holy Grail. Or if you're a spiritual seeker of a more adventurous bent, head up to the third floor to contemplate John Singer Sargent's elegant, yet somber mural sequence *Triumph of Religion.*

One caveat: Library staff urges patrons to never leave their belongings, especially electronics, unattended.

⌣ essentials

✉	700 Boylston Street, Boston, MA 02116
✆	(617) 536-5400
🌐	bpl.org
$	Free
🕐	Monday–Thursday, 9 a.m.–9 p.m.; Friday–Saturday, 9 a.m.–5 p.m.; Sunday (mid-October–May): 1–5 p.m.
🚇	**T:** Green Line, any train, to Copley

peaceful place 7

BEACON HILL STROLL

Beacon Hill, Boston (MAP TWO)

CATEGORY ⌣ enchanting walks ✪

*B*rick sidewalks, working gaslights, and charming 19th-century row houses make a stroll around Beacon Hill like being transported back to a gentler, more elegant time. The antique stores, boutiques, and decor shops on Charles Street provide a refreshing diversion, and the Beacon Hill Hotel's cozy fireplace bar is particularly welcoming on a chilly day. However, I find that an unhurried walk along the Hill's less-trafficked streets is pleasant most anytime.

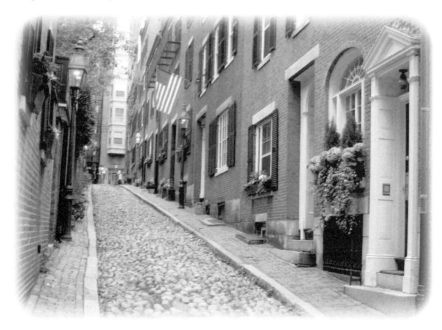

The cobblestone passages and gaslights of Beacon Hill

Upper Mount Vernon and Chestnut streets are where you'll find the Hill's most celebrated architecture: the Federal-style mansions designed by Charles Bulfinch in the early 1800s. (The picturesque yet atypical one-story buildings between 50 and 60 Mount Vernon were originally the stables for the elegant dwellings on the next block, at 13, 15, and 17 Chestnut Street.)

Of course, you'll want to linger a bit in Louisburg Square. For many, this cobblestone street surrounding a large, central private garden epitomizes Beacon Hill. The neighborhood's charming Christmas Eve tradition of carolers, bell ringers, and windows filled with candlelight originated here in the 1860s.

Branch Street, which runs between Charles and Spruce, rewards you with occasional glimpses into some of the neighborhood's famous hidden gardens. And be sure to meander down Cedar Lane Way and block-long Acorn Street, the latter with cobblestones and diminutive houses. Those dwellings were built for the coachmen whose employers lived in the mansions on either side.

This peaceful outing can't help but leave you intrigued by what it might have been like to live in one of these exquisite homes. The well-appointed museum in the circa 1804 Nichols House Museum—with its beautiful furnishings, antiques, and collection of works by the noted Beaux Arts sculptor Augustus Saint-Gaudens—gives you a taste of upper-class 19th-century family life. (The last owner, Rose Standish Nichols, resided here 1885–1960.)

Other intriguing Beacon Hill sights include the House of Odd Windows at 24 Pinckney Street, and Holmes Alley, at the end of Smith Court between Joy and South Russell streets. Holmes Alley is said to have been one of the hiding places for fugitive slaves during the abolitionist era.

Smith Court was the center of Boston's African American life in the first part of the 19th century and is part of the Black Heritage Trail, which celebrates the history of this community. Here, you can pause to explore the Boston campus of the Museum of African American History. The exhibits in the 1835 Abiel Smith School, the nation's first publicly funded schoolhouse for African American children, offer a fascinating counterpoint to the 19th-century opulence you've experienced on the other side of the Hill. I've been eagerly awaiting an opportunity to return to the 1806 African American Meeting House, described as the oldest extant black church building in the United States built by free African American artisans. Closed for the past 4 years while undergoing a $9.5 million restoration, the Meeting House—as this book goes to press—is scheduled to reopen in December 2011, the 205th anniversary of its inauguration. On previous visits, I've found it to be a wonderfully evocative spiritual haven, and I look forward to experiencing that again.

⌣ essentials

▤ **Beacon Hill:** Bounded by Charles, Beacon, and Cambridge streets, Boston, MA 02108 and 02114
Nichols House Museum: 55 Mount Vernon Street, Boston, MA 02108
Museum of African American History: 46 Joy Street, Boston, MA 02114

☏ **Nichols House Museum:** (617) 227-6993
Museum of African American History: (617) 720-2991, ext. 214

🌐 nicholshousemuseum.org
afroammuseum.org/boston_campus.htm

$ **Nichols House Museum:** Adults and children age 13 and older: $7; children 12 and younger: free
Museum of African American History: Adults: $5; seniors age 62 and older: $3; children ages 13–17: $3; children age 12 and younger and members: free

🕐 **Nichols House Museum:** April 1–October 31: Tuesday–Saturday, 11 a.m.–4 p.m.
November 1–March 31: Thursday–Saturday, 11 a.m.–4 p.m. Tours run every 30 minutes.
Museum of African American History: Monday–Saturday, 10 a.m.–4 p.m.
Closed January 1, Thanksgiving, and December 25

🚍 **T:** Green Line, any train, to Arlington or Park; Red Line to Park or Charles/MGH

peaceful place 8

BELLE ISLE MARSH RESERVATION

East Boston (MAP SEVEN)

CATEGORY ↙ outdoor habitats ✪ ✪

oston's largest remaining salt marsh, the 241-acre Belle Isle Marsh provides a hint of what the coastline looked like when the first European settlers arrived on this shore. This is not to say that a visit to the salt- and freshwater marshland protected at Belle Isle will make you feel as though you've left modern-day civilization behind. Houses ring the outer boundary of the reservation on three sides, and Blue Line trains rattle along the remaining edge. Logan Airport sits close enough that, depending on the direction of the wind, planes may thunder by overhead on a regular basis.

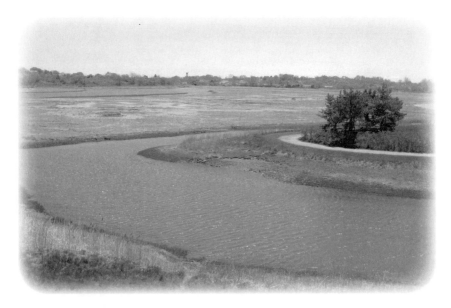

The marshlands at high tide

However, none of that diminishes the serene beauty of this place. The scents of the sea and brackish marsh mingle, and time is told by tides and the birds that make their homes here: shorebirds and songbirds in summer; waterfowl and raptors in winter.

On weekends, Belle Isle Marsh beckons as an enticing family destination, where dogs can roam and kids can ride their bicycles or scooters on the relatively well-maintained gravel pathways. Other times, you may have the place to yourself.

The observation blind offers a panoramic view of the marsh, giving you a peek at the ocean beyond. With a birding scope, you can look out over the salt pans for egrets and ducks. At high tide, you can put in a canoe or kayak and be a part of the rhythms of the marsh. Just about anywhere you wander on warm days, you'll feel surrounded by butterflies and birdsong. Amazing for a place just minutes off the T!

essentials

1284 Bennington Street, Boston, MA 02128

(617) 727-5350

mass.gov/dcr/parks/metroboston/belleisle.htm
friendsofbelleislemarsh.org

Free

Daily, 9 a.m.–sunset

T: Blue Line to Suffolk Downs

peaceful place 9

BOSTON ATHENÆUM

Beacon Hill, Boston (MAP TWO)

CATEGORY ↶ historic sites ✪ ✪ ✪

*A*sk people to name some peaceful places in Boston and they're sure to mention the Boston Athenæum, even though they may never have been there. Such is the reputation of one of the city's most heralded institutions. There's only one catch: as a membership library, the Athenæum—which boasts more than 600,000 books, plus a significant collection of art, sculpture, manuscripts, and maps—permits nonmembers to visit only the rooms on the first floor. However, if you want to experience one of Boston's truly landmark spaces, you shouldn't let this stop you.

Founded in 1807, the library was housed in numerous locations in downtown Boston until 1849, when its collections were moved to this stately building at 10½ Beacon Street. In that era, and for many years after, the Athenæum was the exclusive purview of Boston's most prominent families, with membership shares handed down through generations. No wonder walking through the building's bright red doors can seem a little intimidating at first. (Today, the Athenæum welcomes members regardless of social pedigree.) While visitors are encouraged to take a tour (Tuesday and Thursday at 3 p.m.; reservations required), those who prefer a more solitary excursion are welcome to wander off on their own, pretty much throughout the entire first floor, with the exception of the newspaper room.

The first thing you'll notice is the absolutely stunning view of the Granary Burying Ground, the city's third-oldest cemetery. Savor the undisturbed interior beauty as you move slowly from room to room. Everywhere you look is a treasure. Jean-Antoine Houdon's busts of Benjamin Franklin, the Marquis de Lafayette, and George Washington originally belonged to Thomas Jefferson.

New acquisitions are regularly displayed in the Bow Room, while the Norma Jean Calderwood Gallery hosts three special art exhibitions a year. Don't miss the delightful children's library with its books, toys, and fish tank. Who knows? If you're lucky, maybe you can even find a member who will escort you to the magnificent reading room on the fifth floor.

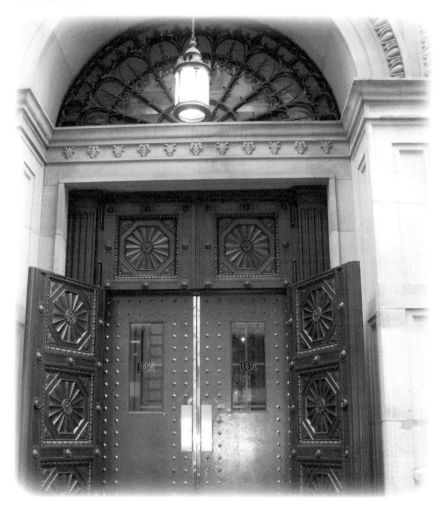

The Athenæum's distinctive doorway

✌ essentials

⊡   10½ Beacon Street, Boston, MA 02108

☏   (617) 227-0270

🌐   bostonathenaeum.org

$ Free, though suggested donation of $5 for entrance to exhibitions

🕐   Monday–Wednesday, 9 a.m.–8 p.m.; Thursday–Friday, 9 a.m.–5:30 p.m.; Saturday,
       9 a.m.–4 p.m.; closed holidays, the day after Thanksgiving, and
       December 24; closes at 5:30 p.m. the day before Thanksgiving

🚊   T: Green Line, any train, to Park Street

peaceful place 10

BOSTON COMMON, FROG POND SKATING

Boston Common, Boston (MAP TWO)

CATEGORY ⌣ outdoor habitats ✪ ✪

*A*s someone who grew up appreciating the pleasures of outdoor skating, I'm a huge fan of the Frog Pond ice rink. Set in the heart of the Boston Common, the Frog Pond serves as a children's wading pool in summer, but from mid-November through mid-March, it's a place where people of all ages can experience the calming effects of gliding effortlessly over glasslike ice. (That is, as long as you can avoid thinking about the possibility of a spill!)

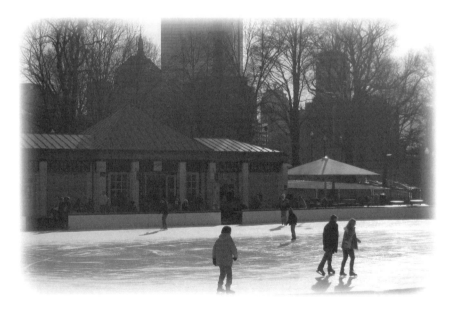

On the ice at the Frog Pond

If you don't own skates, no worries: rentals are available. You can even rent a locker to keep your belongings safe while you indulge your inner Dorothy Hamill or Brian Boitano. Predictably, weekends are the busiest time, so if it's peacefulness that you are after, avoid those days, when the rink is filled with young families and groups of teenagers, many of whom seem to be trying the sport for the first time.

Those with a little more experience might find the weekday early morning freestyle sessions more to their liking. Go when the rink opens at 7:45 a.m., and it's just you, the ice, and the early morning sky, along with a few seasoned skaters practicing their lutzes and Salchows.

For a serene, Currier and Ives–type winter experience, I recommend coming in the early evening, when most people are heading home to supper. As the sun sets, the moon rises, and the stars come out, you'll feel as though you're on a secluded pond instead of in the middle of a big city.

Hot chocolate, sandwiches, and snacks are available at the Frog Pond Café, where you can grab a table and watch the world glide by. For those who are so inclined, the venerable Skating Club of Boston offers group skating lessons.

ﾍ essentials

≡· Boston Common, near 84 Beacon Street, Boston, MA 02108

🕻 (617) 635-2120   🌐 bostonfrogpond.com

$ Adults: $4; children age 13 and younger: free; season passes available; **freestyle sessions:** $12; **adult skate rentals:** $9; **children skate rentals:** $6; **locker:** $2

🕐 **Mid-November–mid-March: Public skating:** Monday, 10 a.m.–4 p.m.; Sunday and Tuesday–Thursday, 10 a.m.–9 p.m.; Friday–Saturday, 10 a.m.–10 p.m. **Freestyle sessions:** Tuesday–Thursday, 7:45–9:45 a.m. Closed Thanksgiving and December 25. Visit website for hours on other holidays.

🚍 **T:** Green Line, any train, to Boylston or Park; Red Line to Park; Silver Line, SL5, to Boylston

peaceful place 11

BOSTON HARBOR ISLANDS NATIONAL PARK

Boston Harbor (MAP FOUR)

CATEGORY ↵ outdoor habitats ✪ ✪

*P*rior to their designation as a national park in 1996, the Boston Harbor Islands were not easy to visit unless you had your own boat. Today, 12 of the 34 islands and peninsulas are easily accessible by ferry. A refreshing island getaway can be yours in as little as 15 minutes from downtown Boston. As the seagull flies, you're never really far from the city. Yet the moment you round Castle Island and head for the outer harbor, time seems to slow down.

Spectacle Island—a former garbage dump that has been reshaped into a terraced mound with two hills, thanks to dirt from the Big Dig tunnel project—is closest to Boston. Though the visitor center and inviting little swimming beach can be bustling on weekends, regular events such as island yoga, jazz concerts, and sunset clambakes will get

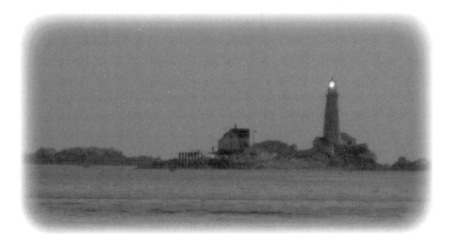

Little Brewster Island and Boston Light

you into a relaxed mood. If you're searching for seaside solitude, there are secluded spots for picnicking along the walking trails to the south and north drumlins, plus some pretty spectacular scenery on the way to the top and back.

Looking for more of a wilderness retreat? Four of the islands—Lovells, Peddocks, Bumpkin, and Grape—have campsites to rent for a night or longer. This is rustic camping, with no flush toilets, no showers, and no electricity or water. However, with any luck, you'll be rewarded with tranquil stargazing and stunning harbor sunrises.

The park service runs trips out to Little Brewster Island's Boston Light from summer into early fall. There, you'll likely be welcomed by Sally Snowman, the 70th in a line of lighthouse keepers there, going back to 1716. (Boston Light is the only remaining Coast Guard–staffed lighthouse in the country.) If you're intrepid enough, you're welcome to climb the 76 steps and two ladders to the top of the lighthouse for a glimpse of the Fresnel lens and the spectacular views. Or you can just gaze out to the Hull shoreline from Ben's Bench, the driftwood chair crafted by a previous keeper, and slowly savor the outer harbor's sights, sounds, and delectable salty smells.

⌣ essentials

📧 **Boston Harbor Islands Pavilion:** On the Rose F. Kennedy Greenway between Faneuil Hall and Long Wharf, 191 Atlantic Avenue, Boston, MA 02110

📞 (617) 223-8666   🌐 nps.gov/boha; bostonharborislands.org

$ **Ferry:** Adults: $14; seniors age 65 and older: $10; children ages 3–11: $8; children age 2 and younger: free; family (two adults and two children): $39.
Boston Light Tour: Adults: $41; seniors age 65 and older and active military: $37; children ages 3–11: $31; children age 2 and younger: free.

🕐 **Ferry schedule:** bostonharborislands.org/ferry-schedule.
Boston Light Tour: June–Labor Day: Friday–Sunday, 10 a.m. and 1:30 p.m.
After Labor Day–late September or early October: Friday and Sunday, 10 a.m.; Saturday, 10 a.m. and 1:30 p.m.

🚇 **T:** Blue Line to Aquarium

peaceful place 12

BOSTON HARBORWALK, DOWNTOWN TO NORTH END

Wharf District, Boston (MAP THREE)

CATEGORY ↲ enchanting walks ✪ ✪

*O*ne might have expected that, as luxury hotels, office buildings, and condo developments spread into the downtown Wharf District, public open space along the water's edge would have disappeared.

Instead, thanks to city officials, environmentalists, and other activists who waged many long and courageous battles, there are more places for strolling and savoring spectacular water views than ever before. Slowly but surely, the Boston HarborWalk is making the dream of being able to walk (or bicycle) almost the entire length of Boston Harbor a reality—taking you all the way from Deer Island in the north, through East Boston and Charlestown, to Boston wharves and Fort Point Channel, and then past the South Boston and Dorchester beaches to the Neponset River in the south.

I'm particularly fond of the HarborWalk section that stretches the 1-mile distance between the Coast Guard Station on Commercial Street to Seaport Boulevard at Atlantic Avenue, with its fountains, plantings, and strategically positioned benches. Here, you can meander amid the sounds of waves lapping against pilings, sailboat halyards clanging in the breeze, and docks creaking in rhythm with the waves.

In the summer and on weekends, some sections can get a little congested, particularly near the aquarium and Christopher Columbus Park. Usually this can be avoided by heading north from Commercial Wharf instead of south. Stretching beyond in that direction, the wharves Lewis, Sargent's, Battery, and Burroughs attract fewer tourists, and the pace is much less hurried.

At Battery Wharf, be sure to listen for the wind chimes, which have been pitched to sound like sailboats' bells. And don't miss the "firehouse" on Burroughs Wharf, where the fireboats Marine Units 1 and 2 are stationed. (It's probably the only firehouse in the country located in a condominium building.)

In warmer weather, The Terrace at the Fairmont Battery Wharf Hotel beckons with harborside tables and seasonal New England fare. (For an experience that's high on nostalgia, if not always peaceful, The Terrace offers marshmallow-toasting kits on Friday and Saturday evenings, so guests can sit around one of the open fire pits and make their own s'mores, evoking the tranquil time of childhood, perhaps.)

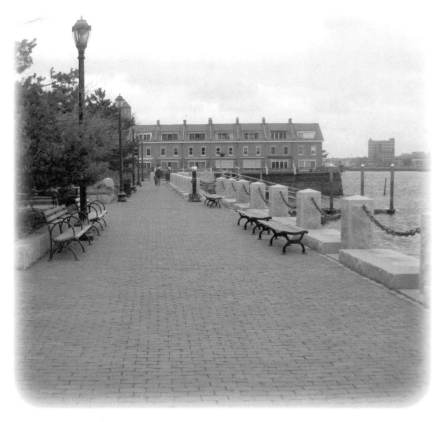

A crowd-free HarborWalk scene

⚲ essentials

⬚ Off of Commercial Street from Burroughs Wharf to Christopher Columbus Park and
Atlantic Avenue from Northern Avenue to Lewis Wharf, Boston, MA 02109 and 02110

☎ (617) 482-1722

🌐 bostonharborwalk.com

$ Free

🕐 Open 24/7

🚌 **T:** Green Line, any train, to North Station; Red Line to South Station; Blue Line
to Aquarium

peaceful place 13

BOSTON MARINE SOCIETY AND SHIPYARD PARK

Charlestown, MA (MAP SEVEN)

CATEGORY ⌣ reading rooms ✪ ✪ ✪

*W*alk into the Boston Marine Society's headquarters at the Charlestown Navy
Yard and you feel as though you've slipped into the realm of a secret society.
Founded as the Fellowship Club in 1742, the society is the oldest association of sea captains in the world.

Currently, there are more than 300 members who remain faithful to the society's
mission of providing for local mariners in need, as well as protecting the safety of Boston

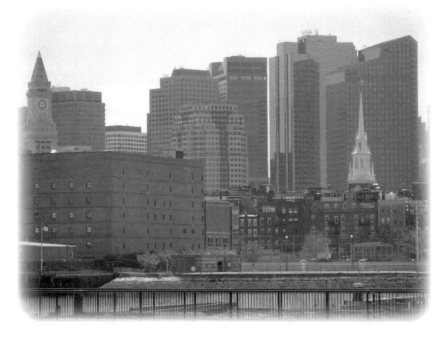

The view toward Boston from Shipyard Park

Harbor. In fact, the Marine Society was responsible for the reconstruction of Boston Light on Little Brewster Island in 1783, having lobbied to replace the one destroyed during the American Revolution 7 years before.

Browsing through the main room's artifacts—including nautical instruments, prints, ship models, and maps—provides a pleasant escape. Except for those rare times when the members are meeting, you're welcome to curl up in one of the comfortable red leather chairs in the library with any of the hundreds of books on maritime history, navigation, and other nautical subjects that members have donated over the years. Want to delve even deeper into Boston's nautical lore? The USS Constitution Museum and the grand ship herself are both located nearby.

Across the street, the beautifully landscaped Shipyard Park offers secluded spots for picnicking, as well as two children's play areas, a fountain for cooling off on hot days, and the impressive Korean War Memorial, where at the touch of a button, you can lose yourself in stories recounted by veterans in their own voices.

Shipyard Park also makes an excellent place to begin an exploration of the Harbor-Walk segments along the water in Charlestown. The panoramic vistas extend from the North End to the Seaport District and beyond. There are waterfront cafés where you can partake of refreshment along with the scenery; at regular intervals, narrative markers chronicle the role that shipbuilding and immigration played in Charlestown's history.

For those who'd like to admire the views from the *water*, the T's water taxis ply the harbor between the Harborview dock and Long Wharf.

essentials

Building No. 32, Charlestown Navy Yard, Charlestown, MA 02129

(617) 242-0522   bostonmarinesociety.org; nps.gov/bost

$ Free   Monday–Friday, 9 a.m.–4 p.m.

T: Inner Harbor Ferry F4 to Charlestown Navy Yard

peaceful place 14

BOSTON NATURE CENTER AND WILDLIFE SANCTUARY

Mattapan, MA (MAP EIGHT)

CATEGORY ↩ outdoor habitats ✪ ✪

ince 2002, Mass Audubon has operated the Boston Nature Center and Wildlife Sanctuary as an environmental conservation and education center, This site enables visitors to leave the city behind and immerse themselves in the wonders of nature. Located on 67 acres at what was once the site of the Boston State Hospital, the Nature Center provides an oasis where you can wander along 2 miles of trails, taking you past wetlands, woodlands, meadows, and fields.

Considering that you're in the heart of a densely populated part of the city, there's a surprising amount of nature: more than 170 species of birds and 46 species of butterflies—in addition to foxes, coyotes, rabbits, and raccoons—have been spotted here. (After a fresh snowfall in winter, it's a great place for kids, and perhaps their adult companions, to learn to identify animal tracks.)

One of my favorite walks is on Fox Trail, a 0.5-mile loop around the wetlands. A short way down this quiet trail, you'll find a welcoming bench where you can rest and listen to redwing blackbirds and yellow warblers and watch dragonflies darting over the marsh. A little farther along is the Andrew M. Kendall Wetlands Overlook Boardwalk, which extends out into the marsh. It's a great place to pause with binoculars or a sketchbook and enjoy the natural sights and scents. If you walk farther, don't be surprised if you catch a whiff of autumn vegetation, even in summer: the city's leaf-composting center is located nearby.

Before or after your walk, be sure to stop by the visitor center in the George Robert White Environmental Conservation Center. It's a showcase for the latest green building technologies, including advanced insulation, passive solar heating and lighting, and geothermal heat pumps.

⌣ essentials
_____

⊞ 500 Walk Hill Street, Mattapan, MA 02126   ☎ (617) 983-8500

🌐 massaudubon.org/Nature_Connection/Sanctuaries/Boston

\$ **Mass Audubon members:** free; **suggested donation for nonmembers:** $2

🕐 **Trails:** Daily, sunrise–sunset. **Nature Center:** Monday–Friday, 9 a.m.–5 p.m.;
Saturday, Sunday, and holiday Mondays, 10 a.m.–4 p.m.

🚌 **T:** Orange Line to Forest Hills or Red Line to Ashmont, then Bus 21 (Ashmont/Forest
Hills Station) to intersection of Morton and Harvard streets

peaceful place 15

BOSTON PUBLIC LIBRARY COURTYARD

Back Bay, Boston (MAP ONE)

CATEGORY ◡ urban surprises ✪ ✪

can always tell when someone has discovered the courtyard at the Boston Public Library for the first time. Usually the person stops and stares in amazement at having stumbled upon this tranquil oasis in the midst of the Back Bay. The arcaded promenade that surrounds the courtyard on three sides is said to be an almost exact replica of the loggias at the Palazzo della Cancelleria in Rome. The sound of water cascading from the courtyard's statuary fountain, a replica of Frederick William MacMonnies's *Bacchante and Infant Faun,* muffles not only the distant street noise but also the sounds of nearby conversations. It is a good place to get lost in a good book or your own thoughts.

I enjoy visiting right after the library opens in the morning. You can grab a coffee from the Map Room Café and write, read, or surf the Web at one of the café-style tables that line the promenade. (The library's free Wi-Fi works here.) At lunchtime on a nice day, when it's hard to find a seat, a table at the library's Courtyard Restaurant provides a pleasant alternative. Note that the restaurant also serves an elegant afternoon tea. Perhaps my favorite time to linger here is in the evening when most people have left for the day. Then the courtyard's subtle lighting produces a soft glow as you watch the sunset colors blaze and then fade in the sky overhead.

Note: Library staff urges patrons to guard their belongings, especially electronics.

◡ essentials

	700 Boylston Street, Boston, MA 02116		(617) 536-5400
🌐	bpl.org		
$	Library courtyard: free; Courtyard Restaurant entrées: $12–$18; Tea: $22.50		

🕐 **Library:** Monday–Thursday, 9 a.m.–9 p.m.; Friday–Saturday, 9 a.m.–5 p.m.; Sunday (mid-October–May): 1–5 p.m. **Courtyard Restaurant:** Monday–Friday, 11:30 a.m.–2:30 p.m. Tea: Wednesday–Friday, 2–4 p.m.

🚌 **T:** Green Line, any train, to Copley

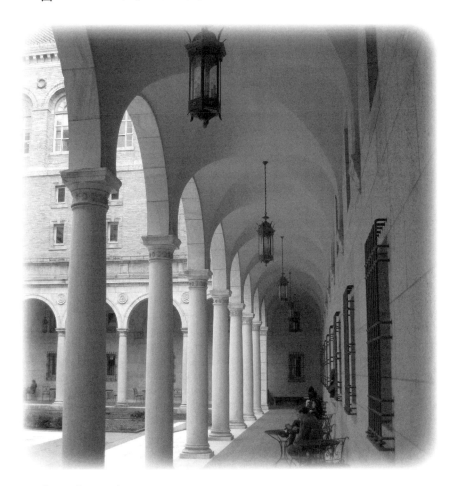

A tranquil courtyard moment

peaceful place 16

CAFE 939, BERKLEE SCHOOL OF MUSIC

Back Bay, Boston (MAP ONE)

CATEGORY ⌣ urban surprises ✪

C afe 939's Red Room is one of the most intriguing music venues in the city. Run by students from the Berklee School of Music, this hip yet comfortable space offers an eclectic range of music by everyone from emerging Berklee artists to local performers to national and international stars looking for a space that enables them to truly connect with their audience.

While the evening shows are justifiably popular, and frequently sold out, I'm a big fan of the free lunchtime gigs held at 1 p.m. most Tuesdays and Thursdays throughout

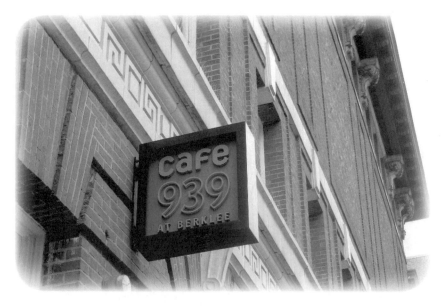

Cafe 939's location in a historic building that dates from 1902

the school year. Depending on the schedule, you may be hearing the improvisations of a solo jazz pianist, an avant-garde faculty group trying out some new pieces, or a rock band playing music from their latest CD. In the spring, the concerts take on a nostalgic tone as the Red Room becomes a venue for final senior recitals by soon-to-be graduates, any one of whom, given Berklee's track record, could turn out to be a future Grammy winner.

For the best experience, I recommend that you get to the Red Room early, so you can sit in one of the comfortable red faux-leather banquettes that line two sides of the room. You're welcome to bring something from Cafe 939. Either way, you'll feel as if you stole away to a swank supper club in the middle of the day and, as you return to your busy life, you may find yourself whistling a happy new tune.

essentials

⌑ 939 Boylston Street, Boston, MA 02115

☎ (617) 747-6038

🌐 cafe939.com

$ Free–$12; varies by performance

🕐 **Café:** Monday–Tuesday, 7:30 a.m.–9 p.m.; Wednesday–Friday, 7:30 a.m.–11 p.m.; Saturday, 10:30 a.m.–11 p.m.; Sunday, 10:30 a.m.–9 p.m.

🚌 **T:** Green Line, B, C, or D train, to Hynes Auditorium

peaceful place 17

CAMBRIDGE CENTER GARAGE ROOF GARDEN

East Cambridge, MA (MAP SEVEN)

CATEGORY ⌣ urban surprises ✪ ✪

*T*he gently curving brick pathways lined with evergreens, birches, and ornamental crab trees are a feast for the eyes. Almost everywhere you look, there are abundant beds of day lilies, lady's mantle, and other perennials that bloom from spring until fall. With benches for reading, tables for picnicking, and substantial patches of lush green grass for lounging or napping, you have ample choices for how to spend your time. And, oh yes,

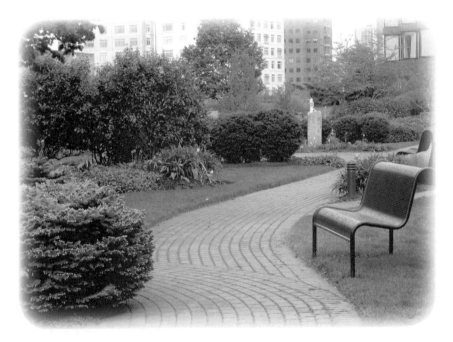

A secret garden six stories above street level

the views of Boston and Cambridge are sublime. That's because this tranquil little garden is six stories above street level, on the top of the otherwise nondescript Cambridge Center parking garage, next to the Boston Marriott Cambridge. Who knew?

This rooftop oasis was once one of the area's best-kept secrets; now that it is better known, it can be teeming with sun-seeking office workers at lunchtime. But otherwise, it's often relatively deserted. If I worked in this neighborhood, I'd stop by on my way to the office for a few yoga stretches on the grass, followed by a little rooftop cappuccino. But you might consider bringing a blanket, a good book, some sunscreen, and water, and settling in for some serious R & R. And keep your eyes open for unusual birds: a pair of falcons is rumored to live atop the Marriott's Residence Inn across the way. *One note:* As the young trees are still small, deep shade is somewhat limited, so it can get pretty hot up here on sunny days when there's no breeze.

∽ essentials

=•   4 Cambridge Center, Cambridge, MA 02142

✆   n/a

🌐   cambridgecenter.info (Click on "Building Amenities" and then "Gardens and Parks.")

$ Free

🕐   Daily, sunrise–sunset

🚃   **T:** Red Line to Kendall/MIT

peaceful place 18

CHARLES RIVER GONDOLA RIDE

Back Bay, Boston (MAP ONE)

CATEGORY ✒ urban surprises ✪ ✪ ✪

*W*hile it may seem surprising to see a boatman plying the waters of the Charles River in the prow of an authentic Venetian gondola, it's not as out of place as you might think. Arthur Shurcliff, the landscape architect who designed the lagoons, islands, and footbridges that give the Charles River Esplanade its distinctive character, was inspired by the canals of Venice.

No doubt he would heartily approve of the tours that Gondola di Venezia has been offering on the Charles since 2001, thanks to a Boston couple who, during their courtship in the 1990s, fell in love with the idea of bringing gondolas to Boston.

Indeed, the slow pace of a gondola ride, accompanied by the sound of water lapping against boat and oar, plus some well-chosen recordings of Italian love songs, is one of the most romantic and tranquil ways to see the city from the water.

Though a daylight cruise is extremely picturesque, a trip near sunset or just after dusk is absolutely magical. The sounds and stresses of city life seem to evaporate as you venture out in solitude onto the hushed river, lit only by the gondola lantern and perhaps the moon. Two people can cuddle in the cushy upholstered seats, but should you want to share the ride with friends, there's room for four more. Wineglasses and a small picnic of cheese, crackers, and chocolates are provided. (The Champagne is up to you.)

The gondoliers excel at pampering their guests. They know how to be solicitous but unobtrusive. They are said to have witnessed many hundreds of marriage proposals, without ever hearing a "no." But you don't have to be celebrating anything that momentous to treat yourself to a gondola ride. A simple yearning for a respite of pure bliss is more than enough.

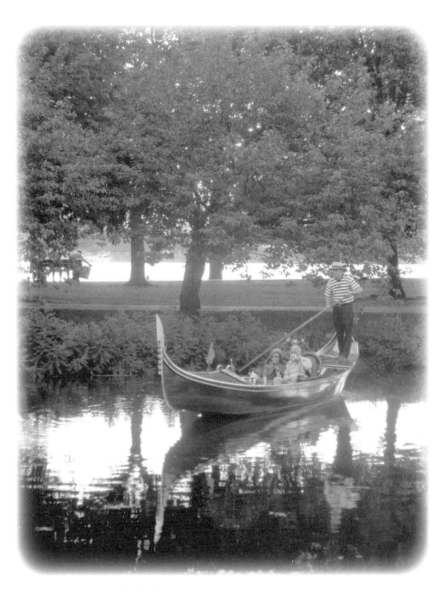

A romantic sojourn on the Charles

essentials

✉	Esplanade near the Hatch Shell, 1 David G. Mugar Way, Boston, MA 02116
☎	(800) 979-3370
🌐	bostongondolas.com
$	$99–$229
🕐	Late May–mid-October, Friday–Sunday, 2–11 p.m. (advance tickets only)
🚌	**T:** Green Line, any train, to Arlington; Red Line to Charles/MGH

peaceful place 19

CHARLES RIVER KAYAKING

Cambridge and Auburndale, MA (MAP SEVEN: SEE 19A; MAP EIGHT: SEE 19B)

CATEGORY ⌣ scenic vistas ✪ ✪

*A*s you float through the water, the tensions of the day seem to dissipate with the breeze and the rhythmic sound of your paddle steadily pushing you forward. While the cities of Boston and Cambridge line the opposite shores, urban life seems small and far away. Instead, the river appears huge and welcoming, and if you keep away from the ubiquitous Boston Duck Tours (which have their place), it's very peaceful.

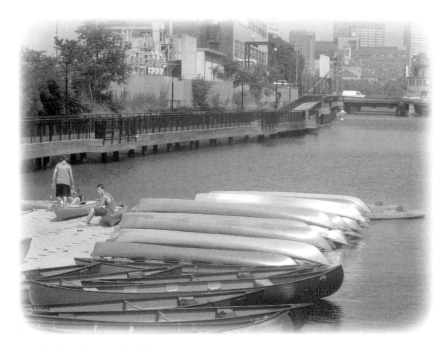

Kayak rentals at the Broad Canal

Thanks to the public boat launch on the recently restored Broad Canal and the rentals offered there through Charles River Canoe & Kayak at Kendall Square, a relaxing paddle along the Charles is more accessible than ever. And it makes for a wonderful escape.

Between the Museum of Science and the Boston University Bridge (see 19A, Map Seven), there's a 9-mile stretch of water to explore, including the tranquil lagoons and canals around The (Charles River) Esplanade. Don't worry here about tides or currents, though a brisk wind can kick up a little wave action. Charles River Canoe & Kayak also offers a one-way trip up the river past the Harvard campus to Herter Park on Soldiers Field Road, and also guided tours of Boston Harbor.

The public launch is free for those with boats. Otherwise you can rent one by the hour, half day, or day. If you work in the vicinity, an early evening paddle could be a refreshing way to put the cares of the office behind you.

If urban kayaking doesn't appeal to you, you might consider the Lakes District, a 6-mile stretch that runs from Auburndale to the Moody Street Dam (see 19B, Map Eight). There are two ways onto the river there: the public boat launch at the Norumbega Duck Feeding Area on the left bank of the river—great if you have your own kayak—and the Charles River Canoe & Kayak's Newton/Auburndale location on the right bank.

This quiet, wooded stretch of river is one of my favorites. It's wide and usually calm, and it is a great place for spying wildlife such as herons, ducks, and turtles, as well as for admiring autumn colors, come fall. And for the ultimate in blissful serenity, Charles River Canoe & Kayak offers a 3-hour moonlight paddle here; it begins as the sun sets over the river and the full moon begins to rise.

⌣ essentials

Broad Canal public launch ramp and Charles River Canoe & Kayak at Kendall Square rentals: 500 Broad Canal Street, Cambridge, MA 02142
Norumbega public launch: 2 Norumbega Road, Weston, MA 02493
Charles River Canoe & Kayak Auburndale tours and rentals: 2401 Commonwealth Avenue, Auburndale, MA 02466

(☎) **Charles River Canoe & Kayak:** (617) 965-5110

(🌐) **Charles River Canoe & Kayak:** paddleboston.com

$ **Public launches:** free; **Charles River Canoe & Kayak:** $15 per hour for a single kayak–$112 per day for a quad kayak

(🕐) **Public launches:** May–October: Daily, sunrise–sunset;
Charles River Canoe & Kayak: weather permitting
At Kendall Square: May–October 23: Saturday–Sunday and holidays, 9 a.m.–30 minutes before sunset. May–Columbus Day: Thursday–Friday, noon–30 minutes before sunset. June–Labor Day: Monday–Wednesday, noon–30 minutes before sunset
At Auburndale: April 1–late November: Saturday–Sunday and holidays, 9 a.m.–30 minutes before sunset; Monday–Friday, 10 a.m.–30 minutes before sunset

(🚌) **Broad Canal in Cambridge: T:** Red Line to Kendall/MIT; **Auburndale:** n/a

peaceful place 20

CHINATOWN PARK

Chinatown, Boston (MAP THREE)

CATEGORY ✦ parks & gardens ✪

hinatown Park was the first of the Rose F. Kennedy Greenway spaces to be completed. However, because it's located some distance from the main stretch of parkland, it's rarely visited by anyone other than locals and nearby office workers.

Built on what was once an abandoned off-ramp for the old Central Artery, this pocket park's bamboo wall screens it from the chaotic traffic beyond, making it almost invisible

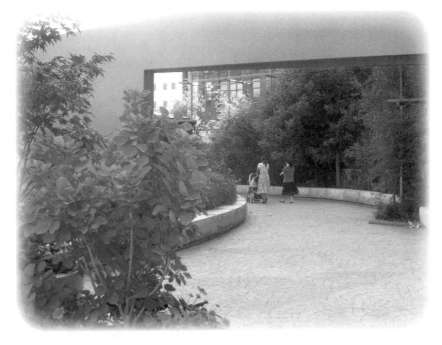

Taking a walk through the red gate into Chinatown Park

to those walking or driving by. While you can enter the park from the main plaza just past the Chinatown Gate at Beach Street, I prefer the more secluded entrance by the striking red gate on the Essex Street end.

A serpentine path leads through a small garden oasis of rhododendrons, cherry trees, peonies, grasses, and other Asian-inspired plantings to a soothing waterfall and stream. I feel that there's a soulful sound that rises from these water features. Perhaps that's because they were created out of stones that once lined the seawalls of the wharves where Asian immigrants arrived in Boston. Kids and adults alike find it relaxing to pause here and dangle their legs into the rushing water, while the noise of the surrounding city disappears.

I find this to be a restorative spot to savor a late takeout lunch from one of the nearby restaurants. There's a calming sense of repose and beauty here, amid all the symbols of balance and harmony. I especially like to contemplate the paving stones, which are laid in a pattern that evokes the scales of a dragon stretching the length of the park. Look for that when you come here.

⌣: essentials

160 Kingston Street, Boston, MA 02228

(617) 292-0020

rosekennedygreenway.org (Click on the "Visit" drop-down menu, then on "Greenway Parks," and then on "Chinatown.")

$ Free

Daily, 7 a.m.–11 p.m.

T: Red Line to South Station

peaceful place 21

CHRISTIAN SCIENCE CENTER REFLECTING POOL

Back Bay, Boston (MAP ONE)

CATEGORY ↙ scenic vistas ✪ ✪

*W*hile you might not expect an open space in the middle of a city to be truly peaceful, the reflecting pool on the plaza at the Christian Science Center should change your mind.

The plaza is sheltered from street noise by buildings on two sides and by a parklike expanse featuring three perfectly spaced rows of meticulously manicured linden trees on the Huntington Avenue side. (Walking under those trees always makes me feel as though I've just been magically dropped into the Jardin des Tuileries in Paris.)

Part of what makes the pool so strikingly unique is its very size. At 690 feet, it's nearly the length of two football fields. In width, it's about half a small city block. The pool's edges are made of curved, polished granite that not only creates a gentle sound as the water laps against it but also fosters the impression that the buildings, trees, and people walking on the opposite end are emerging from the pool. While there are no benches next to the pool, the nearby concrete planters—filled with a profusion of shrubs, grasses, and perennials such as Perovskia (Russian sage), 'Autumn Joy' sedum, and baptisia— were conveniently built to seat height.

The pool becomes a particularly contemplative spot at the end of day, when sunset colors and city lights seem to dance on the water. The strategic placement of the planter benches offers an illusion of privacy from others nearby. For reasons both economic and environmental, the powers that be at the Christian Science Center want to reduce the size and depth of this pool and create a promenade across the middle. It would be very sad indeed to have anything compromise the serenity of this magnificent, singular space.

At the far east end of the plaza is a huge walk-in fountain where children play on hot days. (On days when the fountain is not open due to inclement weather, there is usually a very apologetic sign promising that the fountain will be open as soon as weather improves.) When kids are playing, this part of the plaza may not be peaceful, but it sure is joyful.

essentials

📧   175 Huntington Avenue, Boston, MA 02115

📞   (617) 450-2000

🌐   christianscience.com/church/the-mother-church/boston-activities

$ Free   🕐   Open 24/7

🚌   **T:** Green line, E train, to Prudential or Symphony

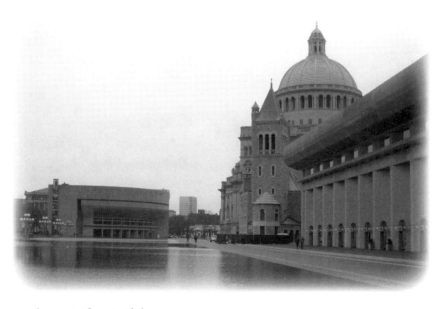

A serene spot for contemplation

peaceful place 22

CITY SQUARE PARK

Charlestown, MA (MAP SEVEN)

CATEGORY ⌣ parks & gardens ✪

*C*ity Square Park looks as though it's been there since Charlestown was founded in 1628, but the truth is that it wasn't built until 1996, after the elevated roadways that had long blemished the neighborhood's center were put underground. Though it takes up just an acre, the park has a magnificent fountain, numerous sculptures, plaques, and memorials, as well as more than 70 varieties of trees, shrubs, and perennials.

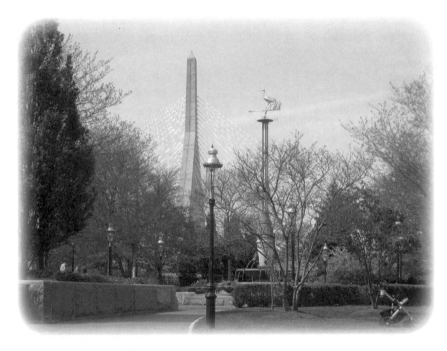

A peaceful moment in City Square Park

Thanks to meandering paths and a strategic use of landscaping, there are places where you can feel as if you've gotten away from it all, despite the park's small size and proximity to busy roads. Authentic working gaslights add to the overall impression of tradition and tranquility. (It's particularly picturesque on foggy evenings.)

If the park is not crowded, I like to sit on the wall opposite the fountain for a great view of the Leonard P. Zakim Bridge in the distance. There, the whoosh of the water muffles any distracting noises.

Elsewhere, be sure to pause by the medallion honoring Elizabeth Foster Goose, who was born in Charlestown and has been called the American Mother Goose—courtesy of the book of her nursery rhymes and fairy tales published by her son-in-law, Thomas Fleet. (Mrs. Goose's grave is one of the most-visited sites in the Granary Burying Ground in Boston.)

Other famous Charlestown residents honored here with medallions are John Harvard and Charles Tufts, founders of the universities that bear their names.

essentials

Bounded by Main Street, New Rutherford Avenue, Chelsea Street, and City Square, Charlestown, MA 02129

n/a

citysquarepark.org

Free

Daily, sunrise–sunset

T: Green Line, any train, or Orange Line to North Station

peaceful place 23

CODMAN ESTATE

Lincoln, MA (MAP NINE)

CATEGORY ↜ historic sites ✪ ✪ ✪

*D*own a quiet lane in Lincoln, not too far from Henry David Thoreau's beloved Walden Pond, lies the historic Codman Estate. Built in 1735–1741 by a wealthy farmer named Chambers Russell, the house and surrounding grounds passed into the Codman family in 1790. With only a few decades' interruption from 1807 to 1862, members of that clan were in residence here until 1968.

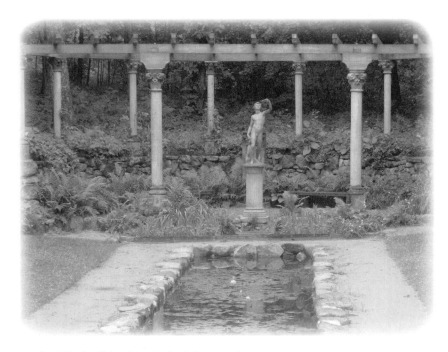

Sarah Bradlee Codman's captivating Italianate garden

For history buffs, the art, furnishings, mementoes, and bric-a-brac on display at The Grange, as the Codmans called their estate, provide a fascinating look at the way the family's interests and tastes evolved over four generations. But the spot I find most enticing is the secluded, Italianate sunken garden that Sarah Bradlee Codman created in 1899–1901.

With its marble-columned pergolas, Greek-inspired statuary, and reflecting pool brimming with water lilies, the garden exudes a tranquil yet haunting air that encourages contemplation. The neatly manicured lawns on either side of the pool make an inviting place to sit with a book or enjoy a picnic. Or perhaps you might prefer one of the stone benches nestled among the ferns and other greenery where the garden meets the woodlands. Here, you can sketch or be lulled into a reverie by the songs of pewees, vireos, and thrushes, undisturbed by visitors who might venture by.

While the house can be seen only during limited hours June–October, the grounds, which also include a meadow and pond, as well as a charming cottage garden designed by Sarah's daughter Dorothy, are open year-round. Lincoln conservation land abuts the property, which means that a visit here can be combined with a walk or bicycle ride in the picturesque countryside.

essentials

34 Codman Road, Lincoln, MA 01773 (617) 994-6690

historicnewengland.org/historic-properties/homes/codman-estate

$ **Garden:** free; **House:** Adults: $5; seniors: $4; students: $2.50;
Historic New England members and Lincoln residents: free

Garden: Daily, sunrise–sunset. **House:** June 1–October 15: Second and fourth Saturdays, 11 a.m.–5 p.m.; tours on the hour with last tour at 4 p.m.

T: Commuter Rail, Fitchburg Line, to Lincoln; then a 0.5-mile, 12-minute walk

peaceful place 24

COMMONWEALTH AVENUE MALL

Back Bay, Boston (MAP ONE: SEE 24A AND 24B)

CATEGORY ↵ enchanting walks ❂ ❂

*D*esigned in 1856 by Arthur Delevan Gilman, the Commonwealth Avenue Mall quickly became a favorite place for Back Bay gentry to promenade. Today, a stroll down the nine-block-long, 100-foot-wide expanse offers an enchanting experience in every season. During summer, the maples, lindens, sweet gums, and American elms create a shaded, cathedrallike canopy that provides a cool oasis for reading or people-watching. For a week or so in mid-April, the mall is the perfect spot to delight in the captivating sight (and fragrance!) of magnolia trees in full bloom along the south-facing side of the street. Come fall, if the weather hasn't been stormy, the trees display their colors deep into November. But the mall is at its most magical early December–late March when approximately 200,000 tiny white lights, wrapped around the trunks of trees, illuminate the pedestrian walkway.

To me, the perfect time to visit is near dusk, which near December's winter solstice can be as early as 4 p.m. A weekend is best, when street traffic declines. If a light snow is falling, so much the better.

Start at the western end, by Charlesgate. Check out the figure of Leif Eriksson, one of nine statues and memorials that decorate the mall. Cross Massachusetts Avenue and continue east. At 314 Commonwealth Avenue, pause and admire the circa 1899 Burrage Mansion, with its limestone griffins, gargoyles, and cherubs. (New England Patriots quarterback Tom Brady used to live in a condo here.)

Now, cross over to the mall. In the next two blocks, look for my favorite statues: between Gloucester and Fairfield, you will come to the *Boston Women's Memorial,* honoring Abigail Adams; Lucy Stone, the abolitionist and suffragette; and African American poet Phillis Wheatley. Between Fairfield and Exeter, you will see the memorial to historian and Rear Admiral Samuel Eliot Morison, with his likeness perched on a rock and gazing seaward.

Along the way, look up into the light cast from residential windows for glimpses of how today's Back Bay denizens live. When you get to Arlington Street, cut through the Public Garden and head to the Bristol Lounge at the Four Seasons Hotel and warm up over a hot chocolate or toddy.

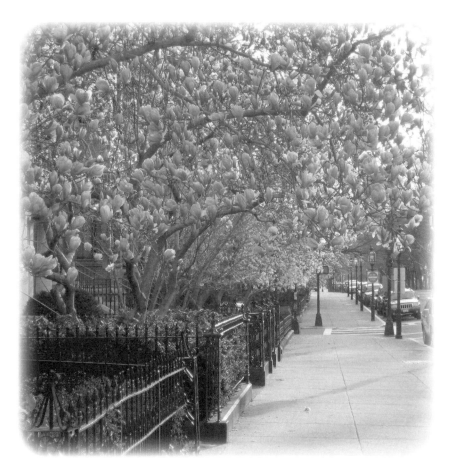

Magnolia trees in bloom on Commonwealth Avenue

essentials

⊡   Commonwealth Avenue between Charlesgate and
      Arlington Street, Boston, MA 02116

Ⓒ   **Friends of the Public Garden:** (617) 723-8144

🌐   friendsofthepublicgarden.org

$ Free

🕓   Open 24/7

🚋   **T:** Green Line, B, C, or D train, to Hynes Auditorium

peaceful place 25

CONDOR STREET URBAN WILD

East Boston (MAP SEVEN)

CATEGORY ⌣ outdoor habitats ✪ ✪

*F*rom Colonial times until the late 20th century, commercial or industrial interests captured most urban rivers and harbor areas in greater Boston, and members of the public rarely ventured there. (The lower Charles River, with its esplanade and canals, marks the one exception.) But happily, that trend is changing, and this once-gritty stretch of land along the East Boston side of Chelsea Creek is a perfect example.

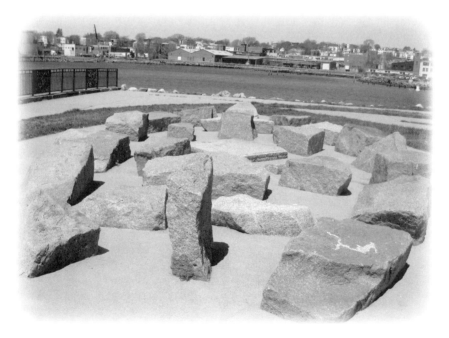

Chelsea Creek Clipper, *a contemporary sculpture formation by B. Amore*

Formerly a brownfield, the 4.5-acre naturalized Condor Street Urban Wild has winding paths that you can follow down to a pier that stretches out into the creek. (Though I've never been lucky enough to see them, rumor has it that this is a great spot for spying harbor porpoises in winter and spring.)

In the distance you will see the tanks that hold jet fuel for Logan Airport, but here you're surrounded by a restored salt marsh and meadow naturalized with river birch, oak trees, Amelanchier, and abundant grasses. On breezy days in the summer and fall, the latter make it appear as if the entire park is swaying in time with the wind. Strategically placed benches provide nice spots to rest and gaze out across the water.

For many people outside of East Boston, coming here may seem too far off the beaten path. Yet there's something alluring about the unusual spirit of this place. The granite monuments at the park's edge tell the stories of some who call this neighborhood home, and their tales are well worth reading.

↲ essentials

☰ Between Condor and Glendon streets, Boston, MA 02128

☎ (617) 482-1722

🌍 bostonharborwalk.com/placestogo

$ Free

🕓 Daily, sunrise–sunset

🚌 **T:** Blue Line to Maverick, then Bus 11, 116, or 117 to Condor Street

peaceful place 26

COPLEY PLAZA HOTEL OAK ROOM

Back Bay, Boston (MAP ONE)

CATEGORY ∿ quiet tables ✪ ✪

*F*or years, Boston wasn't much of a breakfast town. Outside of the big hotels, there weren't many places to find a weekday breakfast that went beyond the basic toast, eggs, and home fries. Nowadays, that has changed, and there are plenty of spots to meet with friends or clients over an early morning repast. But sometimes I yearn for one of those fancy, unhurried hotel breakfasts. That's when I head to the elegant Oak Room at the Copley Plaza (officially known as the Fairmont Copley Plaza).

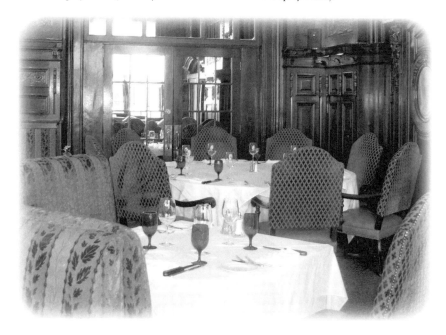

Sumptuous elegance in the Oak Room

Designed by the architectural firm that did both New York's Dakota apartment building and Plaza Hotel, the Copley Plaza has the look of an ornate wedding cake. The lavish, mirrored lobby and ballroom with their gilded ceilings and trompe l'oeil paintings hint of Versailles. In the Oak Room, however, with its dark wood paneling, elaborate window treatments, and stuffed deer heads, the atmosphere is more like that of an English manor.

For greatest serenity, request a booth table. Though the breakfast menu has all the expected items, this is definitely the spot to indulge in some extravagance. For me, that means the New England Benedict, where the traditional eggs are topped with a generous amount of steamed lobster. (I think the accompanying home fries—crispy on the outside, soft on the inside, with caramelized onions and chopped parsley—are the best in the city.) If possible, plan your Oak Room escape for sometime around the holidays, when the lights, greenery, and other decorations add a festive note to your quiet-table retreat.

Note: The dress code is business casual—no sports pants, shorts, T-shirts, caps, sneakers, or sport sandals, and jeans are not preferred.

essentials

✉	138 St. James Avenue, Boston, MA 02116
☎	(617) 267-5300
⊕	theoakroom.com
$	Breakfast entrées: $13–$29; lunch entrées: $14–$36; dinner entrées: $30–$55; brunch entrées: $10–$29
⏱	Sunday–Thursday, 6:30–11 a.m., 11:30 a.m.–2 p.m., and 5:30–10 p.m.; Friday–Saturday 6:30–11 a.m.; 11:30 a.m.–2 p.m., and 5:30–11 p.m. **Brunch:** Sunday, 11:30 a.m.–2 p.m.
🚇	T: Green Line, any train, to Copley; Orange Line or Commuter Rail to Back Bay Station

peaceful place 27

COPLEY SQUARE FARMERS' MARKET

Back Bay, Boston (MAP ONE)

CATEGORY ↝ shops & services ✪

wice a week, from late spring to just before Thanksgiving, Copley Square is home to one of the premier farmers markets in the Boston area. In addition to an incredible selection of seasonal fruits and vegetables, you can buy artisanal cheeses (the goat cheese sometimes featured on the cheese cart at upscale L'Espalier, described on page 70, is on sale here); homemade cookies and pies; fresh cut flowers; herbs in pots for your windowsill or balcony; fresh eggs; and even locally raised, free-range meat. It's

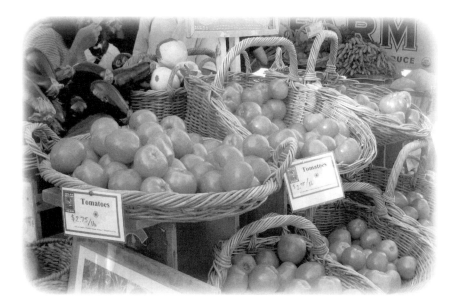

The market's August bounty

not uncommon to find a chef from one of the nearby restaurants picking up some microgreens, berries, or heirloom tomatoes to feature on that night's menu.

Because the market is extremely popular, the trick to ensuring a peaceful experience—not to mention the best selection—is to get here early. Especially if I'm going to pick up some lunch, I try to arrive by 11:30 or so. (The Herb Lyceum makes delightful, out-of-the-ordinary sandwiches, and at the Siena Farms stand, you can find salads, mezes [Mediterranean appetizers], and cold soups from Oleana, one of the top restaurants in the Boston area.)

Once you've completed your shopping, seek out a shady spot near the statue of Phillips Brooks to the north side of Trinity Church. You'll enjoy a respite from the madding crowd yet be close enough for people-watching. On hot days, it's fun to watch kids—and even some adults—splash in the large semicircular fountain.

∾ essentials

[✉] Copley Square, 139 St. James Avenue, Boston, MA 02116

🕜 n/a

🌐 www.massfarmersmarkets.org/fmfm_market1.aspx?mktid=41

\$ Free, except for purchases

🕐 **Mid-May–Tuesday before Thanksgiving:** Tuesday and Friday, 11 a.m.–6 p.m.

🚗 **T:** Green Line, any train, to Copley; Orange Line or Commuter Rail to Back Bay Station

peaceful place 28

D. BLAKELY HOAR SANCTUARY

Brookline, MA (MAP EIGHT)

CATEGORY ⌣: outdoor habitats ✪ ✪ ✪

he D. Blakely Hoar Sanctuary is something of a hidden gem. As you head down Gerry Road, you will be certain that you've wandered into a little suburban neighborhood by mistake. Just as you're ready to give up and turn around, you will see the white entrance arbor and the familiar Brookline nature sanctuary sign. Whew, you've found D. Blakely Hoar!

And once you've begun exploring here, you will know that the trip has been worth it. Because it's a sanctuary, as opposed to a park or conservation land, D. Blakely Hoar

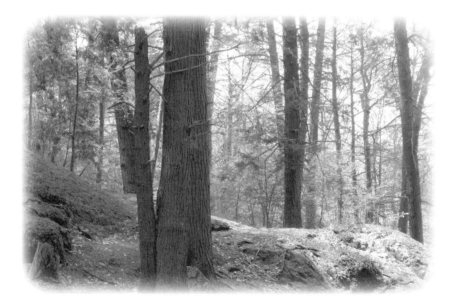

A perfect nature lover's getaway

is more of a tranquil nature refuge than a busy recreation spot. That means that dog walking and activities such as ball playing and bicycling are not permitted here, which makes this the perfect setting for placid pastimes, such as bird-watching, picnicking, or just being one with nature. (Though I haven't tried it, I'm sure that snowshoeing or cross-country skiing would be lovely in winter.)

A trail with three boardwalk areas circles the 25-acre sanctuary. Depending on where you wander, you'll find a wooded upland, wetlands, and, in spring, a vernal pool. The red maple swamp is particularly breathtaking come fall. In summer, the sound of phoebes, pewees, redwing blackbirds, and catbirds fills the air. If you're still, you may spot a wood duck or owl, maybe even a fox or a deer.

D. Blakely Hoar, for whom this restful sanctuary is named, was not the owner of this property but rather the benefactor whose bequest made the purchase possible. It truly is a quiet treasure.

essentials

At Gerry Road, Brookline, MA 02467

(617) 730-2088

brooklinegreenspace.org/pdf/Hoar.pdf

$ Free

Daily, sunrise–sunset

T: Bus 51 (Cleveland Circle/Forest Hills Station) to the Putterham stop

DECORDOVA SCULPTURE PARK AND MUSEUM

Lincoln, MA (MAP NINE)

CATEGORY ↙ enchanting walks ✪ ✪ ✪

While the deCordova Museum is a must-see attraction for art lovers, a visit to its 35-acre Sculpture Park is something between a vision quest and an enticing scavenger hunt for seekers of delightful tranquility. At any given time, this gently rolling landscape of woodlands and lawns contains approximately 75 works of modern and contemporary art, including large-scale sculptures and site-specific

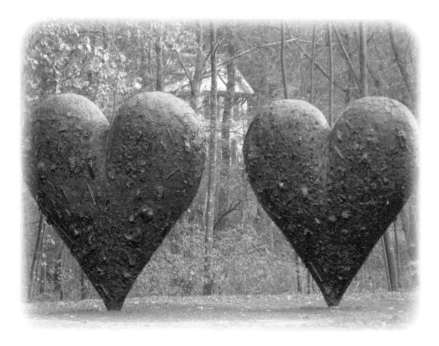

Jim Dine's 1985 sculpture Two Big Black Hearts

installations. But don't worry; there is nothing highbrow about this art scene. Visitors are welcome to roam as they please; you can picnic, walk dogs, and even cross-country ski or snowshoe, if the weather permits. There's only one rule: no climbing on the sculptures. (I find that, given the irresistible nature of much of the work, following that rule always requires a certain degree of self-discipline.)

Organized tours are available, but I prefer simply to wander—with map in hand so I don't miss anything. I like to begin each visit by crossing under the archway of *Rain Gates* at the edge of the parking lot and climbing up through its levels of plantings, stepping-stones, and flowing water. Once in the heart of the sculpture garden, I tend to go where the spirit takes me. Among my favorite sculptures are *Venusvine*, a 16-foot-high bronze goddess that soars into space from its stone perch, and the fascinating *Two Black Hearts*, which you should be sure to visit up close.

Rocks and benches placed strategically throughout the park provide plenty of opportunity to stop, gaze, reflect, or sketch. But keep your eyes open, particularly in Alice's Garden, where smaller pieces surprise at every turn. And don't miss the pinecone figures hidden in the hemlock grove.

When I need a break, I usually head to the museum's Sculpture Terrace for a latte. The Café at deCordova also serves soups, salads, and sandwiches to eat inside, or it can provide the basis for an impromptu alfresco snack amid the garden art.

The park's landscape design itself is a work of art. Nature lovers will appreciate the abundance of beautiful plants and trees that provide interest in every season, as does Flint's Pond at the park's northern edge. (Legend has it that this was the pond that first captured Henry David Thoreau's interest, but he turned to nearby Walden when permission to build a cabin alongside Flint's was refused. If this is true, I can imagine his disappointment.)

I love to linger here near sunset and then return to my car via the Pond Path. Last time, as I stopped to admire the sculpture of a baying wolf, I heard the cry of another predator. Sure enough, a red-tailed hawk glided into view overhead. To me, this living creature heralded the perfect ending to a day of art in the wild.

✎ essentials

✉   51 Sandy Pond Road, Lincoln, MA 01773

☎   (781) 259-8355   🌐   decordova.org

$ **Sculpture Garden grounds, outside of museum hours:** free. **During museum hours:** Adults: $12; seniors and children ages 6–12: $8; children age 5 and younger, museum members, Lincoln residents, and active military and their dependents: free.

🕐   **Grounds:** Daily, sunrise–sunset. **Museum:** Tuesday–Sunday and select holidays, 10 a.m.–5 p.m. **Café:** Tuesday–Friday, 11 a.m.–3 p.m.; Saturday–Sunday, 11 a.m.–4 p.m.

🚌   n/a

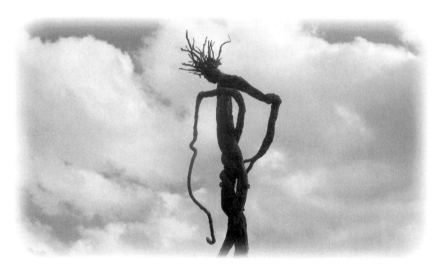

Venusvine by Richard Rosenblum, 1990

peaceful place 30

DORCHESTER HEIGHTS

South Boston (MAP FOUR)

CATEGORY ◡ historic sites ✪ ✪

While not as famous as the midnight ride of Paul Revere, the fortification of Dorchester Heights marked a pivotal moment in the American Revolution. On March 4, 1776, under cover of darkness, George Washington's militia surreptitiously moved 59 cannon to the Heights's summit. Not long after, the British were forced to evacuate their troops and loyalists from the city below, and Boston and its strategic harbor belonged to the colonists. To commemorate that victory, in 1902, a 115-foot white Georgian marble tower was erected there.

Despite the fact that the city has grown up around it, the site, also known as Thomas Park, still enjoys a commanding view of downtown Boston to the north, the Back Bay to the west, and Dorchester and the suburbs to the south.

The twisting, inclined streets and Victorian houses that surround the park remind me a bit of San Francisco. (Ironically, one of those streets is even named Telegraph.) Though the tower is open only in the summer months, the park is a pleasant place to bask in the sun on the grassy areas that face south, or curl up on a bench and read in the shade in one of the far corners. Be warned, though, that it's a popular place for locals to let their pooches run free, so on weekends or at prime dog-walking times, your serenity could be interrupted by some frisky canine fun.

◡ essentials

⌧	Between Telegraph, Old Harbor, and G streets, Boston, MA 02127
☏	(617) 242-5642
☉	nps.gov/bost/historyculture/dohe.htm

$ Free

Park: Daily, sunrise–sunset. **Tower:** Mid-June–August: Call for hours

T: Red Line to Andrew

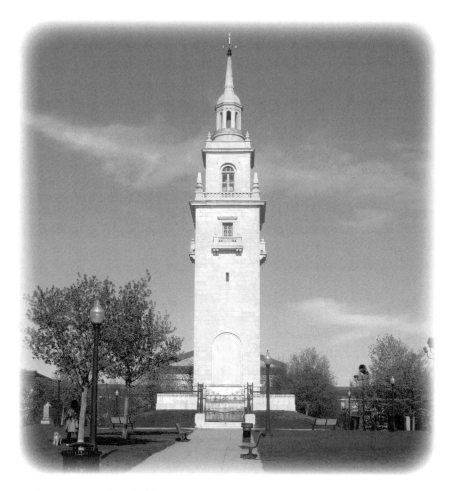

The tower at Dorchester Heights

peaceful place 31

L'ESPALIER SALON

Back Bay, Boston (MAP ONE)
CATEGORY ↻ quiet tables ✪

I'm sure that most people have favorite restaurants that they return to again and again for special occasions. Since the late 1970s, L'Espalier has been one of mine. Though I have fond memories of its former location in an exquisite Back Bay townhouse, the swank digs adjacent to the Mandarin Oriental Hotel do offer some advantages. One of these is the elegant, yet welcoming, salon where one can drop in for a drink and light repast after work or an evening's night out.

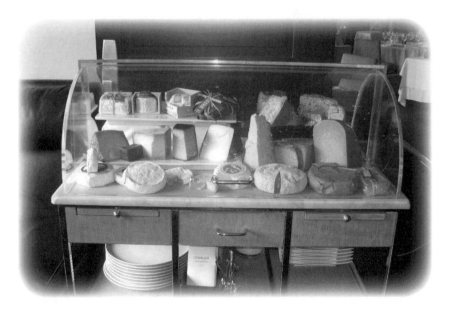

Trolley de fromage *at L'Espalier*

The special salon menu offers an interesting selection of bites, samplers, and plates, as well as signature dishes and desserts. You may also order off the dining room menu, if you wish, though it's a tad pricey. In the salon, I recommend trying one of the cheese flights concocted by *fromagier* and maître d' Louis Risoli. Whether you like your cheese blue, gooey, stinky, or local—or prefer to request your own selection from the abundant *trolley de fromage*—you're in for a treat. You also are likely to sample some varieties you won't find anywhere else.

For optimal serenity in the salon, ask to be seated in the oversize chairs by the windows overlooking Boylston Street. From this comfortable perch, you can luxuriate in the attentive service, tempting tastes, and peaceful Back Bay views.

↲ essentials

774 Boylston Street, Boston, MA 02199

(617) 262-3023

lespalier.com

$ **Cheese flights:** $12.50 small; $25 large. **Other offerings:** $4 bites–$50 grand tasting for two

Monday–Friday, 11:30 a.m.–2:30 p.m. and 5:30–10:30 p.m.; Saturday–Sunday, noon–1:45 p.m. and 5:30–10:30 p.m.
Tea: Saturday–Sunday, 2–3:30 p.m.
Salon: Cocktails and small bites, Sunday–Thursday, 5–10:30 p.m.; Friday–Saturday, 5–11:30 p.m.

T: Green Line, any train, to Copley

peaceful place 32

ETHER DOME, MASSACHUSETTS GENERAL HOSPITAL

Beacon Hill, Boston (MAP TWO)

CATEGORY ↵ historic sites ❂ ❂

*T*he Ether Dome at Massachusetts General Hospital (MGH) gets its name
from the historic operation performed there on October 16, 1846, when W. T. G.
Morton was said to be the first to publicly demonstrate the use of an inhaled anesthetic
on a patient during surgery. From 1821 to 1868, this Charles Bulfinch–designed amphi-
theater was the site of 8,000 operations. (How many of those were performed *before*
the use of anesthetics is something I'd rather not consider, especially when cultivating a
peaceful frame of mind.)

Today, if not in use for medical meetings or lectures, the Ether Dome remains open to
the public. As you walk up the stairs to its fourth-floor location, you'll see encased memorabilia, including early surgical tools and a painting commemorating that landmark
surgery. (According to the hospital's website—because there had been no photographs
taken of the original event—in 2000, some 20 MGH surgeons, physicians, and guests
donned period costumes and reenacted a mock operation to provide the realism that the
artists needed to provide an accurate accounting.)

When you get to the Ether Dome, be sure to say hello to Padihershef, the 2,600-year-
old Egyptian mummy that has been in residence here since 1823, and then find a seat
and take a few minutes to admire this fascinating historical and architectural space. As
long as you don't contemplate what it was like to be a surgical patient here in the early
days, it can actually be quite peaceful to spend some time under the skylit dome.

essentials

⊡ 55 Fruit Street, Bulfinch Building, Fourth Floor, Boston, MA 02114

☎ (617) 726-2862

🌐 massgeneral.org/history/exhibits/etherdome

$ Free

🕐 Monday–Friday, 9 a.m.–5 p.m.; closed during faculty meetings

🚌 **T:** Red Line to Charles/MGH

peaceful place 33

FANEUIL HALL

Quincy Market, Boston (MAP THREE)

CATEGORY ↝ historic sites ✪

he Faneuil Hall marketplace is regularly listed in the top five of the most-visited tourist attractions in America, so it's no surprise that I, like many Bostonians, seldom venture there. In fact, it wasn't until I attended a business function in the meeting hall known as the Cradle of Liberty that I realized just how special Faneuil Hall really is.

The first floor was originally designed as a marketplace; today it serves as a souvenir shop, so it's wise to skip this and go directly to the second-floor meeting hall where

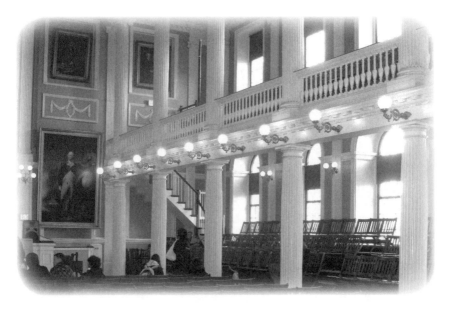

The meeting hall known as the Cradle of Liberty

Samuel Adams and other Boston patriots gave the fiery speeches that inspired the American Revolution. (In actuality, this room was redesigned and enlarged in 1806 by Charles Bulfinch, who added the galleries on three sides of the meeting hall, among other changes. However, the copper-gilded grasshopper weather vane that sits proudly atop the building is the original.) Later years brought installations of paintings that celebrate famous orators who have appeared here, including the somewhat fanciful one of Daniel Webster speaking to an audience that includes George Washington and John Hancock, as well as John Adams and son John Quincy Adams.

Today, Faneuil Hall still plays an important role in the nation's civic life. John F. Kennedy made this the last stop in his 1960 presidential campaign. In 2004, Bostonian John Kerry chose this site for his concession speech in the presidential election that he lost to President George W. Bush. And every other Thursday, a special naturalization ceremony is held here for new U.S. citizens.

While the meeting hall is rarely peaceful due to frequent tours, it's possible to sit off to one of the sides and meditate on the meaning of a place where freedom seems to be in the very air. In the early mornings, particularly in December, the hall can be downright serene.

essentials

1 Faneuil Hall Square, Boston, MA 02109

(617) 523-1300

www.thefreedomtrail.org/visitor/faneuil-hall.html

Free

Daily, 9 a.m.–5 p.m. **Historical talks:** Daily, 9:30 a.m.–4:30 p.m. every 30 minutes. Closed January 1, Thanksgiving, and December 25

T: Blue or Orange Line to State; Green Line, any train, to Government Center

peaceful place 34

FENWAY PARK

Kenmore Square, Boston (MAP FIVE)

CATEGORY ↙ urban surprises ✪

*A*s I walk up Brookline Avenue away from Kenmore Square, I feel a twinge of excitement. There's something irresistible about the prospect of heading into the heart of Red Sox nation, even though it's 9 a.m. and the team is out of town. That's because I'm about to experience a still little-known Boston attraction: the Fenway Park tour.

OK, it's a tour, so there's lots of talk—and too much unnecessary denigrating of the Yankees, in my honest opinion. Yet there's no denying the sense of being on historic, even hallowed, ground. In his famous essay "Hub Fans Bid Kid Adieu," John Updike called Fenway a "lyric little bandbox of a ballpark" where "everything is painted green and seems in curiously sharp focus, like the inside of an old-fashioned peeping-type Easter egg." That's exactly the feeling you get when looking out from the stands at a field empty of everything except a few groundskeepers tending the emerald grass.

Though the tour lasts only 50 minutes, you'll be regaled with fascinating facts and lore. You'll also get to view the park from a variety of different vantage points, including the seats atop the famous left field wall known as the Green Monster and, when the team is away, the press box.

Because there were only 12 of us on my tour, I had plenty of opportunities to sit back and smile as my personal Red Sox highlight reel ran in my head: seeing catcher Carlton Fisk "wave the ball fair," as it's termed, in 1975; learning how to track the game on a scorecard; and watching the eclipse of the moon as the Sox won their first World Series in 86 years.

Early morning tours offer the best opportunity to avoid the crowds. While you may be tempted to wait for the off-season to schedule your visit, you'll miss the magic of seeing the tranquil field of green sparkling in the sun. For those who find it hard to contemplate a trip to Fenway without hearing the crack of a bat, the final tour on game days allows you to stay for batting practice. While it won't be quiet, it definitely will be memorable.

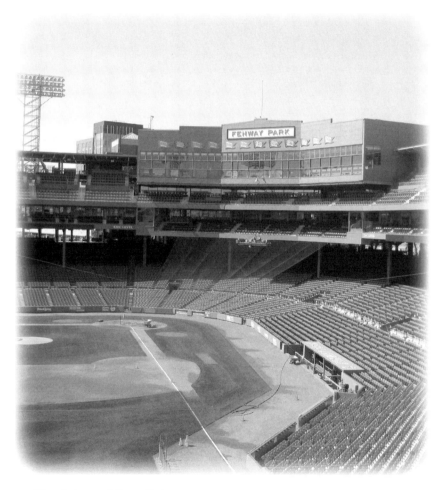

The quiet beauty of Fenway Park

⌣ essentials

⊟   Brookline Avenue at Yawkey Way, Boston, MA 02215

✆   (617) 226-6666

🌐   redsox.com (Search for "tours.")

$ Adults: $12; seniors: $11; children ages 3–15: $10

🕐   Tours: Non-game days: Daily, 9 a.m.–4 p.m. every hour. Game days: 9 a.m.–3½ hours before game time, every hour.

🚋   T: Green Line, B, C, or D train, to Kenmore; Green Line, D train, to Fenway

FENWAY VICTORY GARDENS

The Fenway, Boston (MAP FIVE)
CATEGORY ⌣ parks & gardens ✪ ✪ ✪

$\mathcal{U}$nless there is a game going on at neighboring Fenway Park, the 7-acre Fenway Victory Gardens is a charming oasis, where the only sounds you'll hear are singing birds and buzzing bees. At the height of the flowering season, delightful fragrances fill the air, and it's hard to resist burying your nose in a luscious rose or peony blossom. (Just watch out for the aforementioned bees!)

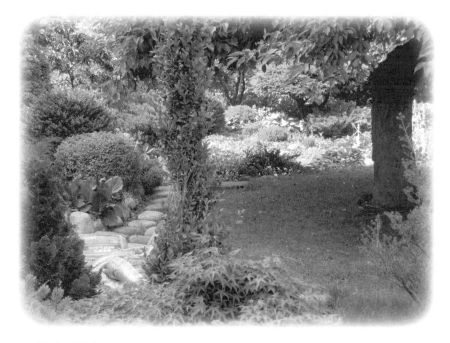

My friend Ricky's garden, among the community plots

During World War II, just about every community in the nation created victory gardens, where locals could raise vegetables to supplement their ration books. The 500 or so Fenway garden plots, each measuring about 15 by 25 feet, are said to be among the only survivors of that era in the nation. Though today you're more likely to find perennials, shrubs, and even dwarf conifers and ornamental trees growing here, I'm sure that bounties of tomatoes and herbs are still cultivated every season.

The gardens are most impressive May–October. While the official entrance to the gardens is at the corner of Boylston Street and Park Drive, I suggest that you enter where Boylston meets The Fenway and stroll along the main walkway, meandering down the side of the plots whenever a particularly interesting garden, unusual plant, whimsical birdhouse, or other ornamental feature catches your eye. Toward the middle of the gardens, you'll find the picnic grounds, where you can spread out a blanket and enjoy a leisurely weekend brunch or sunset supper.

Some gardeners have taken on two, three, or even four plots to create some of the Fenway's most interesting garden displays. You'll want to linger here, admiring the sophisticated plantings and intricate designs with pathways, pergolas, and even a few fishponds.

↵ essentials

✉	Boylston Street at Park Drive to Fenway, Boston, MA 02115
☎	(617) 267-6650
🌐	fenwayvictorygardens.com
$	Free
🕐	Daily, sunrise–sunset
🚊	T: Green Line, B, C, or D train, to Kenmore

peaceful place 36

FOREST HILLS CEMETERY

Forest Hills, Boston (MAP EIGHT)

CATEGORY ↲ enchanting walks ✪ ✪ ✪

eginning in 1848, Forest Hills Cemetery was not only Boston's first public park, but it also functioned as an open-air museum, arboretum, and nature preserve, in addition to being the final resting place of choice for many of the city's most prominent families.

In keeping with the Victorian era's attitude toward death, the entrance gate was designed to give the impression that one was crossing from one dimension—the world of the living—to the other side. Indeed, the 275-acre Forest Hills Cemetery does seem

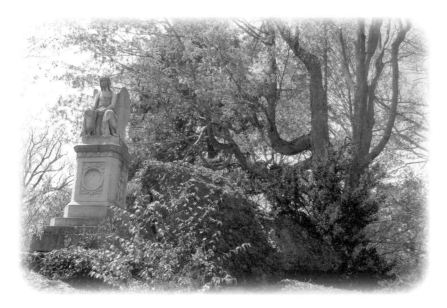

An example of the cemetery's renowned collection of 19th-century memorial sculpture

to have a bit of an otherworldly air. Elaborate memorial sculpture was all the rage from the mid-19th to the early 20th centuries, and Forest Hills boasts a superb collection of masterpieces by some of that era's finest artists and artisans.

If it's your first time here, you may want to pick up a map near the entrance to guide you on a contemplative walk past some of Forest Hill's greatest treasures. One of my favorites, Daniel Chester French's *Angel of Peace,* stands by the grave site of Boston philanthropist George R. White, who also bought the little drumlin across from his plot so he would always be able to look out on nature. Thanks to his foresight, this makes a particularly lovely place to enjoy a picnic. Indeed, in spring, with birdsong and the scent of flowering cherries and crab trees wafting by, you may feel as though you've slipped into paradise yourself! For

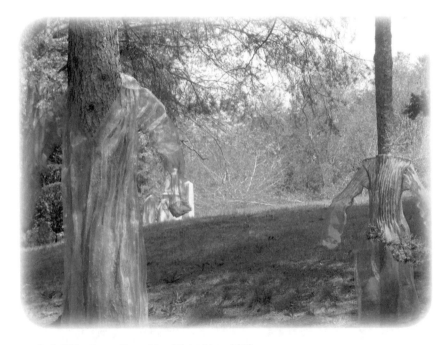

Leslie Wilcox's evocative sculpture Nightshirts, *2002*

those whose taste in art runs to the more modern, the cemetery's contemporary sculpture collection includes more than 30 works from both local and national artists.

Unlike many cemeteries that operate under strict rules of decorum, Forest Hills has a whimsical spirit. For instance, on the gravestone commemorating playwright Eugene O'Neill and his third and final wife, Carlotta Monterey, you'll find stones, tiny good luck charms, and even copies of plays left by admirers.

In another corner of the cemetery, there's a hollowed-out tree where the complete works of e. e. cummings are usually stored in a waterproof bag. The poet himself is buried within sight of that tree, in the plot belonging to his mother's family, the Clarkes. (It strikes me as something of a heresy that cummings's name not only appears, like an afterthought, on the side of the Clarke memorial stone but also was chiseled in capital letters!)

You may want to plan a visit in July for the Annual Lantern Festival. Inspired by a Japanese Buddhist memorial celebration, it offers a tranquil scene, as visitors are invited to share stories and honor loved ones by setting small lanterns afloat in the cemetery's pastoral Lake Hibiscus.

essentials

95 Forest Hills Avenue, Boston, MA 02130

(617) 524-0128

foresthillscemetery.com
foresthillstrust.org

$ Free

Grounds: Daily, sunrise–sunset. **Office:** Monday–Friday, 8:30 a.m.–4:30 p.m.; Saturday, 8:30 a.m.–1 p.m.

T: Orange Line to Forest Hills Station

peaceful place 37

470 ATLANTIC AVENUE OBSERVATION DECK

Waterfront District, Boston (MAP THREE)

CATEGORY ⌣ scenic vistas ✪ ✪ ✪

*F*rom the John Hancock Hotel at Copley Square, to Marriott's Custom House
near the Financial District, to the Foster's Rotunda at the Boston Harbor Hotel at
Rowes Wharf, for one reason or another, many of the places where one could once get a
bird's-eye view of the city have been closed or restricted. That's what makes the observation deck on the 14th floor of Independence Wharf such a treasure. All you have to do

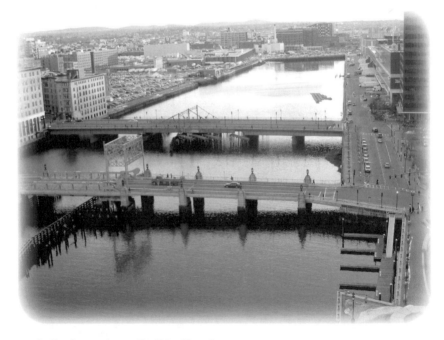

Looking down and across Fort Point Channel

is show a picture ID to the building's security guard and an elevator will whisk you up to a panoramic space that few people know about and even fewer visit.

Walk out onto the viewing area, and you'll hear nothing but the whoosh of the wind and sound of seagulls. (Word to the wise: Sometimes it can be cold and galelike up there, even if it doesn't seem so at ground level, so bring a wrap.) To the south, you'll look out over Fort Point Channel. To the east, you'll have great views of inner Boston Harbor, the airport, and the Harbor Islands. Walk to the west end of the building for views up and down the Rose F. Kennedy Greenway and into the heart of the city. (Some accounts of this space mention a set of stationary binoculars looking out over the waterfront. Don't count on using them; I found them impossible to focus.)

If the weather is pleasant enough, you will want to linger on either of the two benches. Enjoy the sun and sights, and maybe even bring a brown-bag lunch. If it's raining or too chilly, head for the tiny indoor observation room. Hearty souls might want to venture up here in late fall or early winter for stunning views as the sun sets over the city and the lights come twinkling on.

◡ essentials

☰	Independence Wharf, 470 Atlantic Avenue, Boston, MA 02110
☎	n/a
🌐	n/a
$	Free
🕙	Monday–Friday, 10 a.m.–5 p.m.
🚍	T: Blue Line to Aquarium

peaceful place 38

FRANKLIN SQUARE

South End, Boston (MAP FOUR)

CATEGORY ↲ parks & gardens ✪

*E*nclosed by elegant cast-iron fencing, with shaded, tree-lined paths leading to an imposing decorative fountain, Franklin Square (like Blackstone Square, its virtually identical twin across Washington Street) conjures images of Victorian families promenading in all their finery.

The original 1801 Charles Bulfinch design called for a single 5-acre public park here, to be named Columbia Square after the first American ship to circumnavigate the globe. (Bulfinch's family had been investors in that maritime achievement.) However, by the time developers finally got around to realizing Bulfinch's vision, the space had been divided into two uneven parcels by the construction of Washington Street. The result was two parks: Franklin Square, completed in 1849, and its seemingly mirror image, Blackstone Square, completed in 1855.

Today Franklin is considered by some to be a seedier version of Blackstone. The latter does offer a children's play area and dog park, but I prefer Franklin's quieter ambiance. On warm summer days, the shade there seems deeper, and there is ample space for reflection in the far corner where the fountain provides respite from the city sounds.

Franklin Square enjoys notable surroundings well worth exploring: Boston's South End is listed on the National Register of Historic Places as the largest existing Victorian residential neighborhood in the country. A peaceful stroll here can lead you to six other garden squares, most of which feature a central fountain and a cast-iron border. Of these, Worcester Square and Union Park offer the most charm. You'll find the former at the intersection of Harrison Avenue, Washington, and East Springfield and East Concord streets. Union Park, on the street of the same name, is between Tremont Street and Shawmut Avenue. Chester Square, originally conceived as the grandest South End garden square of all, still retains a good measure of its 19th-century character, despite being bisected by Massachusetts Avenue in the 1950s.

✌ essentials

▣ Washington Street between Newton and Brookline streets, Boston, MA 02118

🕐 n/a   🌐 n/a

$ Free   🕐 Daily, sunrise–sunset

🚌 **T:** Silver Line 4 or 5 to Newton Street

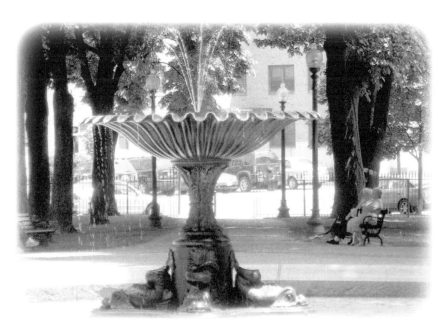

The dolphin fountain at Franklin Square

peaceful place 39

FRENCH CULTURAL CENTER OF BOSTON

Back Bay, Boston (MAP ONE)

CATEGORY ↙ reading rooms ✪ ✪

*O*K, I won't pretend that it's like taking a trip to Paris. But a visit to the French Cultural Center of Boston can be a refreshing break from the typical day-to-day city life here. Relax in the comfortable first-floor reading room, brew yourself a cup of coffee or hot chocolate ($1.50 for nonmembers), and peruse the French version of the latest *Elle* or *Marie Claire*.

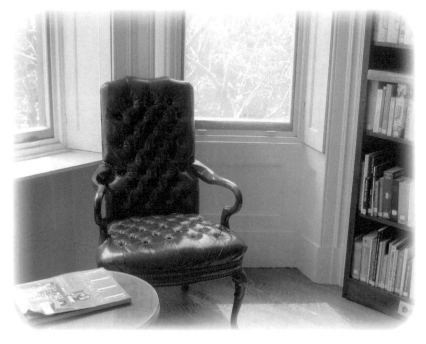

An enticing spot to read

If you'd like to indulge in a little fantasy instead, head to the upstairs library and pull up a chair next to the shelf full of green Michelin guidebooks, and ponder the pleasures of traveling through Normandie or the Haute Savoie—known, respectively, as Normandy and the French Alps to us Americans. In separate areas of the center, you can also brush up on your French by chatting with other visitors or by watching French-language cartoons and cooking shows on TV.

According to the center's website, the library houses the second-largest private collection of French books, periodicals, DVDs, and audio and video cassettes available in the United States. Though only members are allowed to take books and other materials home, the public is pretty much welcome to spend as much time as they wish browsing through the collections—and soaking up the atmosphere of this former Back Bay mansion.

Free Wi-Fi is available for those in search of a quiet work space where English is not the primary language. If you're interested in contemporary French art, the gallery area to the right of the main entrance hosts frequent exhibitions. For those with *les enfants* in tow, there's a bright and cheery children's library with more than 1,000 picture books and storybooks. Come for the morning, or even for just an hour, and feel as though you've had *une petite vacance.*

essentials

✉	53 Marlborough Street, Boston, MA 02116
ℭ	(617) 912-0400
🌐	frenchlib.org
$	Free
🕐	Monday, Tuesday, and Thursday, 10 a.m.–6 p.m.; Wednesday, 10 a.m.–8 p.m.; Saturday, 10 a.m.–5 p.m. Library closed month of August.
🚃	T: Green Line, any train, to Arlington

peaceful place 40

FRUITLANDS MUSEUM

Harvard, MA (MAP TWELVE)

CATEGORY ↙ day trips & overnights ✪ ✪

*F*ruitlands Museum nestles along a ridge that provides a spectacular view across the Nashua River Valley to Mount Wachusett in the west and Mount Monadnock to the north.

The land, including 210 acres of fields, meadows, woodlands, and pine barrens, has a deep spiritual history. Once the hunting grounds of the Makamachekamucks,

Nashua River Valley

it was also a favorite place of Ralph Waldo Emerson, Henry David Thoreau, and other Transcendentalists (visit **transcendentalists.com**). In 1843, Bronson Alcott conducted a brief utopian-living experiment at the Fruitlands Farmhouse with his family—which included 10-year-old Louisa May—and a small group of Transcendentalist followers.

Today, a 3-mile network of trails winds its way through the property. You can choose a brief walk in the woods or take a loop that can occupy an hour or more. Although the trails can be popular on weekends, I've found it to be quite serene; usually all you'll hear is the wind in the trees and the singing of birds. (Nearly 55 species of birds have been recorded here.) Although birding is best in the spring, I think the nicest time for walking is the fall. By then, the biting insects are mostly gone and the maples, cherries, and oaks are in rich, full color. Fruitlands is also a lovely place to experience the hushed sounds of winter on cross-country skis or snowshoes.

For a walk that promises a different type of contemplation, try the museum's spiral fieldstone labyrinth. The design was inspired by the 19th-century Pima basket you can see among the Southwest collection in the museum's Native American Gallery. The gallery houses artifacts from the Plains, Northwest Coastal, and Arctic native tribes. Also on the property is the Fruitlands Farmhouse; an art gallery with a permanent collection of more than 400 pieces, including more than 100 landscapes from the renowned Hudson River School; and the Shaker Office, which was relocated from the Shaker Village in Harvard in 1920.

The museum offers a wide range of special events, outdoor concerts, and lectures. There's also the Alcott Restaurant and Tea Room. Whether you dine inside or under a garden arbor, you can enjoy a lunch or Sunday brunch with a view to soothe your soul.

✌ essentials

⊟ 102 Prospect Hill Road, Harvard, MA 01451

☎ (978) 456-3924, ext. 235

🌐 fruitlands.org

$ **Adults:** $12; **seniors and students with college ID:** $10; **children ages 5–13:** $5; **children age 4 and younger and members:** free. **Trails/grounds only: Adults:** $6; **children:** $3; **members:** free

🕐 **Museum:** Mid-April–mid-November: Monday–Friday, 10 a.m.–4 p.m.; Saturday–Sunday and holidays, 10 a.m.–5 p.m.

🚌 n/a

peaceful place 41

GLOUCESTER STREET DOCK

Back Bay, Boston (MAP ONE)
CATEGORY ↙ scenic vistas ✪ ✪ ✪

*S*cenic vistas beckon along the entire length of the lower Charles River, on both the Boston and the Cambridge banks. So why do I single out the Gloucester Street Dock for special mention? Location, location, location.

Simply by walking down the stairway, you'll leave the commotion of bicycles and joggers behind. Sitting on the dock gives you the sensation of being suspended just above the water level, so you'll feel as if you're part of the river. Look east and get a duck's-eye

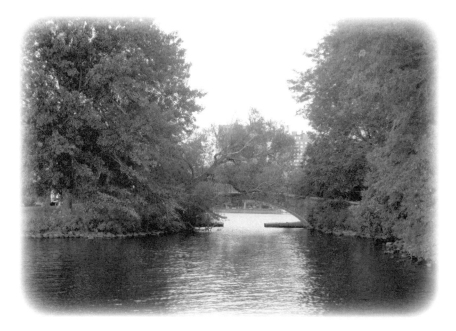

A duck's-eye view of the Charles River lagoon

perspective of the Esplanade lagoon, which was designed to mimic the canals of Venice. Straight ahead is Massachusetts Institute of Technology's Great Dome, frequently the target of clever student pranks called "hacks"—the most famous of which involved a full-size replica of an MIT police car sitting on top of the dome. At sunset, the views to the west can be absolutely awe-inspiring, especially in the fall when the lingering twilight is reflected in the river.

At prime times on sunny weekends, the dock can be less than peaceful, but most times, you can pretty much have it to yourself. Bring a cushion or yoga mat, and sit down with a carryout cup of coffee and your journal. Or simply stretch or meditate. In no time, the background noises disappear and you're breathing with the rhythm of water lapping the shore.

⌣ essentials

✉ Charles River Esplanade between Gloucester Street and Massachusetts Avenue, Boston, MA 02115

☎ (617) 227-0365

🌐 esplanadeassociation.org

$ Free

🕐 Open 24/7, but not recommended at night

� T: Green Line, B, C, or D train, to Hynes Auditorium

peaceful place 42

GREATER BOSTON BUDDHIST CULTURAL CENTER

Cambridge, MA (MAP SIX)

CATEGORY ⌣ spiritual enclaves ✪ ✪ ✪

he facade looks like just another ordinary storefront on one of Cambridge's busiest thoroughfares, but the space inside 950 Massachusetts Avenue has a decidedly spiritual bent. Run by two nuns, the Greater Boston Buddhist Cultural Center (GBBCC) offers a place to feed both body *and* soul.

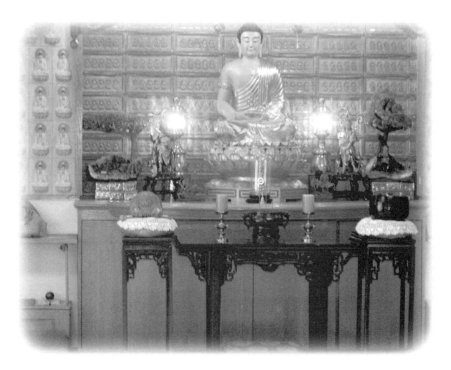

The meditation room at the Greater Boston Buddhist Cultural Center

When you open the door, the scent of incense wafts out to greet you. Straight ahead, as you enter, the library welcomes you to peruse the collection of books on topics from Buddhist philosophy to art history. On the left, the meditation hall provides a hushed space for contemplation, prayer, or simple relaxation. Feel free to take off your shoes, pick up a cushion, and settle into the calm.

For many people, the best part of the GBBCC is the tearoom, where, 5 days a week, you can enjoy a simple yet flavorful four-dish vegetarian meal. For optimum serenity, ask for one of the tables by the window that overlooks the small garden.

Every second and fourth Friday evening, the center hosts a Dinner with Dharma, beginning with a meditation session at 6:30 p.m., followed by dinner and a Dharma talk and discussion.

✑ essentials

950 Massachusetts Avenue, Cambridge, MA 02139

(617) 547-6670   n/a

$ **Tearoom:** Prix fixe lunch: $6.95; **Dinner with Dharma:** Adults: $10; students: $5

Center: Tuesday–Sunday, 11 a.m.–6 p.m. **Meditation Hall:** Tuesday–Sunday, 3–5 p.m.; **Tearoom:** Tuesday–Saturday, 11:30 a.m.–5:30 p.m.

T: Red Line to Central Square

peaceful place 43

GROPIUS HOUSE

Lincoln, MA (MAP NINE)

CATEGORY ↵ outdoor habitats ✪ ✪ ✪

$\mathcal{T}$hose who think of the New England countryside as a place with quaint 17th-, 18th-, and 19th-century villages and farmhouses may be surprised when, driving down Baker Bridge Road in Lincoln, they find themselves passing the white, cubelike home designed by famed Bauhaus architect Walter Gropius.

It was built as the family home in 1938, when Gropius took up a position at Harvard University's Graduate School of Design, and it's said that every aspect of both the house and surrounding landscape were planned for maximum efficiency and simplicity. A visit to the house, which still contains the family's furnishings and art, more than confirms this. But while you can view the house only as part of a tour, there is an alternative: Historic New England, the preservation society that cares for the property, invites visitors to wander and enjoy the 5.5 acres of gardens, meadows, woodlands, and the orchard as you please.

Though the large boulders and mature trees appear to have been placed there by Mother Nature, the Gropiuses themselves are actually the ones who carefully positioned every element of this landscape. (One particularly large boulder situated near the place where the more formal lawn area gives way to the naturalized meadow makes an excellent backrest for a tranquil picnic on the lawn—which is welcome here.)

The small Japanese-inspired garden, designed in 1957 by Ise Gropius (the architect's second wife), is especially lovely in spring when the azaleas and candytuft bloom. As the house is the main draw for most visitors, you are likely to have the grounds to yourself, especially when no tours are scheduled.

This part of the town of Lincoln is also a nice destination for a tranquil stroll or bike ride, as the Lincoln Land Conservation Trust, the Lincoln Conservation Commission, and the Rural Land Foundation of Lincoln have preserved a combined 2,000 acres and more than 70 miles of trails in the area. Maps and trail guides can be purchased by mail or at the Old Town Hall, town offices, or at many local businesses. To learn more, visit **lincolnconservation.org.**

↝ essentials

🖃   68 Baker Bridge Road, Lincoln, MA 01773   📞   (781) 259-8098

🌐   historicnewengland.org/historic-properties/homes/Gropius%20House

\$ **Gardens:** free. **House:** Adults: $10; seniors: $9; students: $5; Historic New England members and Lincoln residents: free

🕐   **Gardens:** Daily, sunrise–sunset. **House:** June 1–October 15: Wednesday–Sunday, 11 a.m.–5 p.m. October 16–May 31: Saturday– Sunday, 11 a.m.–5 p.m. Tours every hour; last tour at 4 p.m. Closed most major holidays.

🚌   n/a

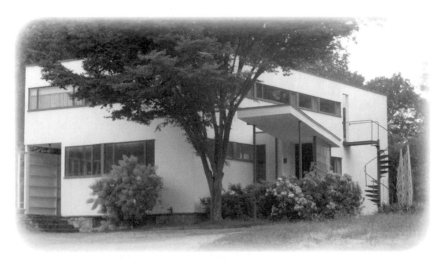

Walter Gropius's famous Bauhaus-style home, built in 1938

peaceful place 44

GUEST HOUSE AT FIELD FARM

Williamstown, MA (MAP TWELVE)

CATEGORY ↝ day trips & overnights ✪ ✪ ✪

*I*t takes about 3 hours to drive from Boston to this one-of-a-kind guesthouse nestled in a valley between the Berkshire Mountains and the Taconic Range, just down a country road from the picturesque community of Williamstown. But once you're there, you'll find all the ingredients for a tranquil weekend getaway.

More than 300 acres of pastures, meadows, and woodlands surround the small inn and its five guest quarters. The lawn, filled with perennial gardens and mod-

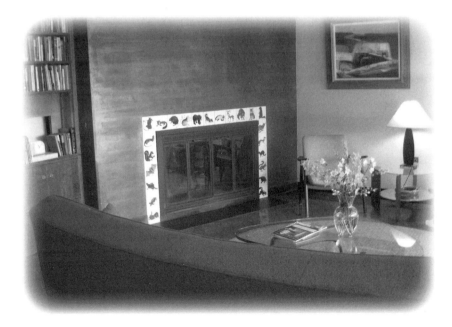

A spot for curling up by the living room fireplace

ern sculpture, overlooks a bucolic pond with views all the way to Mount Greylock, Massachusetts's highest mountain.

Inside the comfortable, circa 1948 modernist house resides a collection of contemporary furniture and artwork lovingly assembled over the years by the former owners, Lawrence and Eleanor Bloedel. Yes, that gorgeous yellow-and-orange painting in the upstairs hall *is* a Wolf Kahn. Of course, that's an original Noguchi coffee table in the living room. (The house and furnishings now belong to the Trustees of Reservations, which has made only minor changes.)

In cool weather, you can relax by a fireplace framed by decorative tiles celebrating the woodland creatures found on the property. (The telescope by the picture window provides an opportunity for you to view the real fauna.) On warm days, you can savor a swim and picnic by the pool. And, just up the road, the store at Cricket Creek Farm sells homemade bread and local cheeses. For a truly luxurious retreat, three of the six guest rooms have private decks, and two of those have fireplaces.

The property also offers 4 miles of public trails for carefree meandering. In early summer, you can delight in the scent of new-mown hay and the soothing songs of bobolinks, meadowlarks, wood thrushes, and veeries. In the fall, the surrounding woodlands, hills, and mountains put on a colorful display.

Of course, no stay in the environs of Williamstown would be complete without a stop at The Clark, as the Sterling and Francine Clark Art Institute is known. Its stunning collection of art from the 15th to the early 20th centuries makes it one of the country's top museums. One caution: Through 2014, a number of The Clark's renowned French Impressionist paintings are on an international tour. Also, area visitors interested in 21st-century art should make time for a visit to MASS MoCA (translation: Massachusetts Museum of Contemporary Art) in North Adams, a sprawling art complex that is transforming that historic factory town.

⌣ essentials

The Guest House at Field Farm: 554 Sloan Road, Williamstown, MA 01267
Sterling and Francine Clark Art Institute: 225 South Street, Williamstown, MA 01267
MASS MoCA: 87 Marshall Street, North Adams, MA 01247

The Guest House at Field Farm: (413) 458-3135
Sterling and Francine Clark Art Institute: (413) 458-2303
MASS MoCA: (413) 662-2111

thetrustees.org/field-farm
clarkart.edu
massmoca.org

$ The Guest House at Field Farm: April and November–December: $150–$275; May–
October: $175–$295. 2-night minimum stay on weekends; 3-night minimum on holidays
and other selected weekends. **Field Farm grounds:** free, though donations appreciated.
Sterling and Francine Clark Art Institute: Mid-October–May: free. June–mid-October:
Adults: $15; members, children age 17 and younger, and students with a valid ID: free
MASS MoCA: Adults: $15; students: $10; children ages 6–16: $5; members and
children age 5 and younger: free

The Guest House at Field Farm: April–December; **Field Farm grounds:** Daily, sunrise–sunset
Sterling and Francine Clark Art Institute: September–June: Tuesday–Sunday, 10 a.m.–
5 p.m. July–August: Daily, 10 a.m.–5 p.m.
MASS MoCA: September–June: Wednesday–Monday, 11 a.m.–5 p.m.
Check for extended hours during holiday weeks in December, February, and April.
July–August: Daily, 10 a.m.–6 p.m.

  n/a

peaceful place 45

GUILD OF BOSTON ARTISTS

Back Bay, Boston (MAP ONE)

CATEGORY ᨳ museums & galleries ✪ ✪

*F*rom the outside, the Guild of Boston Artists has a slightly imposing air, like one of those venerable, members-only institutions that still dot the Back Bay. In actuality, this little-known spot is one of the best places in town to immerse one-self in art from the contemporary realist school.

Established as an artist-owned gallery in 1914, the guild is now an association of approximately 60 painters and sculptors from around New England. The sharp scent of

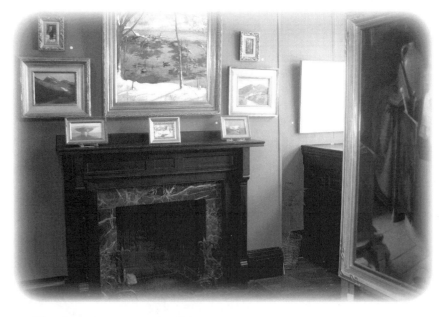

The main viewing area among the galleries

linseed oil and turpentine drifting down from a fourth-floor artist's studio sets the mood and adds a nice touch of authenticity to this salonlike setting. (My mother was an artist, so to me, this smell has an effect similar to Marcel Proust's madeleines.)

While the first room, with its teal walls, has a rather formal feel, the President's Gallery in the rear is a particularly inviting space—perhaps contrary to its name—with a comfortable sofa and coffee table full of art books. The abundant light, courtesy of an impressive skylight that extends over most of the ceiling, is sure to brighten your mood on even the dreariest day. The exhibits change on a regular basis, which makes the guild a refreshing place to unwind. Should you find yourself inspired to try your hand at contemporary realist painting, the guild offers occasional workshops for the public, as well as artists' talks and other events that will steep you in this style of art.

If all this art makes you yearn for more, you might want to extend your artistic excursion a little longer by wandering over to The Copley Society of Art, another artist-owned gallery just a couple of doors away.

essentials

✉	162 Newbury Street, Boston, MA 02116
☎	(617) 536-7660
🌐	guildofbostonartists.org
$	Free
🕐	Tuesday–Saturday, 10:30 a.m.–5:30 p.m.
🚋	**T:** Green Line, any train, to Copley

peaceful place 46

HABITAT EDUCATION CENTER AND WILDLIFE SANCTUARY

Belmont, MA (MAP NINE)

CATEGORY ↵ outdoor habitats ✪ ✪ ✪

*A*s befits a Massachusetts Audubon site, the Habitat Education Center is a haven for birding and for observing native wildlife and flora. (The sanctuary's birding list includes nearly 90 species.) Throughout the 93-acre oasis in this secluded corner of Belmont Hill, a network of trails leads you to meadows and woodlands and by wetlands, ponds, and vernal pools. All render the perfect setting for spring, summer, and fall strolls, as well as for wintertime snowshoeing or cross-country skiing.

Should you prefer a less-active form of recreation, the formal gardens with flowering trees, shrubs, perennials, and expansive lawn areas offer plenty of tranquil places to read, sketch, or nap—or, for children, to play. (Children seem to delight in games of hide-and-seek here, and their happy voices can add to your aural pleasure.) In spring, when the crab apple trees bloom—and again in early summer, when the rose garden is at its peak—the air fills with the most delightful perfume, and birdsong is plentiful. There's also an art gallery in the site's Georgian-style mansion, with regularly changing exhibits of nature-inspired photographs and paintings.

Habitat offers many programs for adults and children throughout the year, so especially during school vacation weeks, there can be a lot of activity. At those times, you may want to venture off to one of my special spots: the Weeks Pond Trail, a short walk away off Somerset Street. The trail crosses a burbling brook and opens out onto a graceful little pond. Choose a bench or, better yet, find a nice flat rock by the water's edge, where, if you're quiet enough, you can catch a glimpse of one of the pond's many amphibian denizens. Alert: In insect season, bug spray is a must at the Habitat!

✌ essentials

⊟ 10 Juniper Road, Belmont, MA 02478

☎ (617) 489-5050

🌐 massaudubon.org/Nature_Connection/Sanctuaries/Habitat

$ **Adults:** $4; **children ages 2–12 and seniors:** $3;
   Mass Audubon members and Belmont residents: free

🕐 **Trails:** Daily, sunrise–sunset. **Visitor center and gallery:** Monday–Friday,
   8:30 a.m.–4:30 p.m.; Saturday–Sunday, 10 a.m.–4 p.m.

🚌 n/a

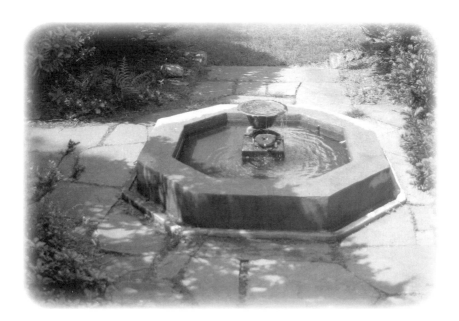

The fountain near the formal gardens

peaceful place 47

HALL'S POND SANCTUARY AND AMORY WOODS

Brookline, MA (MAP EIGHT)

CATEGORY ⌇ outdoor habitats ✪ ✪ ✪

*H*all's Pond Sanctuary is a real treasure: the site showcases a tiny dot of wilderness in the midst of the big city. Yet there's a lot of nature packed into this serene little space. In addition to typical suburban mammals such as squirrels and raccoons, an astonishing diversity of plants and wildlife exists here. On any visit, you are likely to

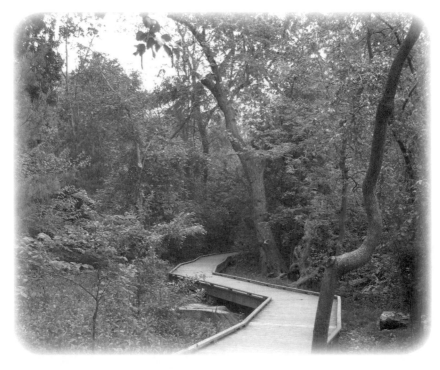

The winding boardwalk trail at Hall's Pond

spot creatures ranging from dragonflies and hummingbirds to painted turtles and garter snakes to herons and cormorants. On early mornings during migration, in the spring and fall, you're almost certain to find warblers singing and calling from the treetops.

The pond is named for the Hall family, who once owned this and much of the surrounding land. (Minna Hall was one of the founders of the Massachusetts Audubon Society.) The sanctuary, at just over 5 acres, consists of a pond, wetlands, uplands, and a wooded section called Amory Woods. While most people use the north entrance beside the parking lot, I recommend coming in via the formal garden at the south entrance, next to the tennis courts. If you're not in a rush, it's the perfect place to linger to read, sketch, or simply admire the plantings of native perennials and shrubs.

The sanctuary's boardwalk trails make it easy to take a peaceful stroll around the pond and wetlands. The upland section, with its bark mulch path, gives the illusion of going deep into the wild, although beautiful homes are just outside the sanctuary to your right. Amid the towering trees in Amory Woods, you'll find some benches and a little gazebo, where someone has inscribed brief excerpts from the writings of Rainer Maria Rilke, Pablo Neruda, Hermann Hesse, and Vladimir Nabokov.

True, it doesn't take long to traverse the paths at Hall's Pond, but I find that after even the briefest respite, I always leave feeling centered and calm.

essentials

Amory Street between Beacon and Freeman streets, Brookline, MA 02446

n/a

brooklinema.gov (Choose "Parks and Open Spaces" from the "Departments" drop-down menu.)

$ Free   Daily, sunrise–sunset

T: Green Line, C train, to Powell

peaceful place 48

HARVARD DIVINITY SCHOOL QUADRANGLE LABYRINTH

Cambridge, MA (MAP SIX)

CATEGORY ↝ spiritual enclaves ✪ ✪

I sometimes think that the path to peacefulness begins with mindfulness. At least that's the way I felt when I first encountered the labyrinth at the Harvard Divinity School Quadrangle. Unlike a maze, which is designed to confuse, the circular path of a labyrinth provides a way to the center and back that's absolutely dependable, though intentionally not direct.

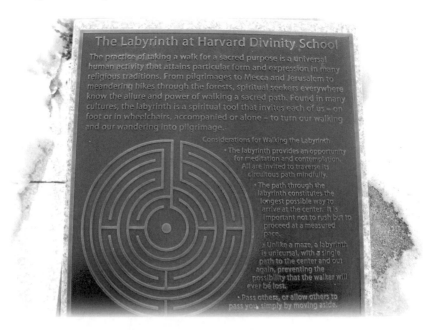

Signage for a mindful path to meditation and contemplation

The Harvard labyrinth is said to be based on a 13th-century pattern from the floor of the Cathédrale Notre-Dame de Chartres, southwest of Paris. As with that intricate course, which has attracted pilgrims for centuries, the one at Harvard is not for lackadaisical strolling. I found that I needed to give my walk my full attention in order to stay on the path. Fortunately, a sign at the entrance to the labyrinth provides instructions as to how to proceed if you meet another walker on your journey within the narrow boundaries, but the day I was there was quiet, except for a few robins singing in the trees.

Labyrinths, which were extremely popular in medieval times, have had something of a renaissance in recent years. A labyrinth is planned for the Armenian Heritage Park on the Rose F. Kennedy Greenway. Boston College also has one, created as a memorial to alumni killed in the attacks on 9/11.

Some people use a labyrinth as a means to deepen meditation and inspire reflection. As I walked Harvard's Divinity School Labyrinth, I kept hearing the words to the Shaker hymn "Simple Gifts" over and over in my mind: "To turn, turn will be our delight, Till by turning, turning we come 'round right."

ى essentials

47 Francis Avenue, Cambridge, MA 02138

n/a

hds.harvard.edu (Search for "labyrinth.")

$ Free

Open 24/7

T: Red Line to Harvard Square

peaceful place 49

HARVARD MUSEUM OF NATURAL HISTORY AND PEABODY MUSEUM OF ARCHAEOLOGY AND ETHNOLOGY

Cambridge, MA (MAP SIX)

CATEGORY ⚬ museums & galleries ✪ ✪

*F*or a double dose of escape, visit both of these adjacent museums whenever you need to get your mind off work, current events, or whatever else plagues you at the moment. Though both are popular, there are ways to avoid the crowds.

But first, a bit of background: Unlike a typical museum, the objects, specimens, and artifacts on display at both the Harvard Museum of Natural History and the Peabody Museum of Archaeology and Ethnology were not originally meant for public enjoyment but rather for serious academic study. Contrary to what you might expect, the natural history museum is one of the Boston area's newest, established in 1998 to bring to a wider audience the collections of three Harvard research museums: the Museum of Comparative Zoology, the Herbaria, and the Mineralogical and Geological Museum.

The natural history museum's most famous collection, the Glass Flowers, is also one of its most popular. (Although rumor has it that some visitors—after viewing these amazingly realistic botanical specimens fashioned from glass, wire, paint, and enamel—will plaintively ask, "But where are the *glass* flowers?") Because the Glass Flowers are so lifelike, I find that a visit to this collection is a particularly restorative sight in winter. Where else would you find desert cacti, tropical orchids, and blue flag irises in bloom at the same time?

Kids, naturally, love the dinosaur exhibits, the large mammals, and the meteorites. (To be honest, so do the adults.) These exhibits can get crowded and noisy, especially on weekends or weekday mornings when school tours drop in. One of my favorite places to escape is to the small balcony located just above Great Mammal Hall, where specimens from Harvard's splendid collection of North American birds are displayed. There I can sit on a bench by a window and sketch some of the beautiful hummingbirds and warblers or just marvel that creatures this tiny and delicate can travel the distances they do on their twice-a-year migrations.

The admission fee to the Museum of Natural History also entitles one to visit the adjacent Peabody Museum of Archaeology and Ethnology, and I like to take advantage of that fact to stop by and see the Alaskan masks and totem pole in the Northwest Coast room of the Peabody. I always find it deeply moving to spend a few silent moments contemplating the stories that these artifacts tell and the secrets that they must hold.

Should you visit when the weather is accommodating, the Boyer Quadrangle, just behind the museums, offers a serene place to enjoy a picnic lunch or just a few calming minutes before you get back to your day.

essentials

Harvard Museum of Natural History (HMNH): 26 Oxford Street, Cambridge, MA 02138
Peabody Museum of Archaeology and Ethnology (PMAE): 11 Divinity Avenue, Cambridge, MA 02138

HMNH: (617) 495-3045; PMAE: (617) 495-2269

hmnh.harvard.edu
peabody.harvard.edu

Adults: $9; non-Harvard students with ID and seniors age 65 and older: $7; children ages 3–18: $6; members and current Harvard ID holders plus one guest: free; Massachusetts residents (with proof of residency): free every Sunday, 9 a.m.–noon and Wednesday (September–May), 3–5 p.m. See website above for additional admission discounts. The Museum of Natural History is adjacent to the Peabody Museum of Archaeology and Ethnology, and admission to one museum admits you to both.

Daily, 9 a.m.–5 p.m.; closed January 1, Thanksgiving, December 24, and December 25

T: Red Line to Harvard Square

peaceful place 50

HARVARD SQUARE BOOKSTORES

Cambridge, MA (MAP SIX)

CATEGORY ⌣ shops & services ✪

*C*all me old-fashioned, but I prefer to browse in a real bookstore, where I can take a leisurely walk, pick up a book in my hand, and voilà!—find something unexpectedly perfect. That's what makes this five-block section of Harvard Square a one-of-a-kind destination you just can't experience with online shopping.

The Harvard Book Store takes up two levels in a high-ceilinged old building that smells deliciously like books. This being Harvard Square, the substantial remainder tables (30%–70% off), feature titles such as *Chinese Brushwork* or *Thousand Mile Song: Whale Music in a Sea of Sound*—rather than Robert Ludlum page-turners or celebrity bios. A solid selection of books avails itself in every category, from architecture to

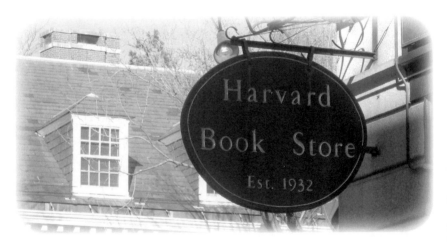

One of an endangered species: an independent bookstore

zoology. I especially like the fact that staff recommendations capture attention on shelves throughout the store.

In comparison to the size of Harvard Book Store, the Grolier Poetry Book Shop is tiny. Reportedly the oldest continuous poetry bookshop in the United States, the Grolier stocks more than 15,000 volumes of poetry, prosody, and criticism, many from small independent publishers or university presses that you will be hard-pressed to find anywhere else.

Like the Grolier, Schoenhof's Foreign Books is a specialty store, offering what is likely the largest selection of foreign books in North America. You'll find everything from

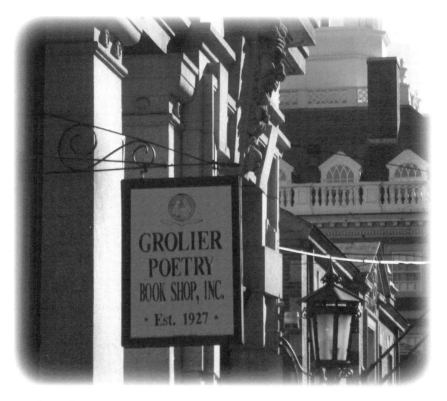

A poetry lover's delight

novels to scholarly works, in nearly a hundred different languages and dialects. There's also a good-size children's section with books in some 11 languages, including Hebrew, Hindi, and Hungarian.

All three stores can get crowded on weekends or when an event is scheduled. But at lunchtime and evenings, you can find yourself pleasantly alone. While it is too small to provide space for reading benches or chairs, the Harvard Book Store does have a secret nook near the Myths, Tales, and Fables section. I like to head for that comfy purple seat, especially when it is dappled with afternoon sun.

✓ essentials

📧   **Harvard Book Store:** 1256 Massachusetts Avenue, Cambridge, MA 02138
       Grolier Poetry Book Shop: 6 Plympton Street, Cambridge, MA 02138
       Schoenhof's Foreign Books: 76 Mount Auburn Street, Cambridge, MA 02138

📞   **Harvard Book Store:** (617) 661-1515
       Grolier Poetry Book Shop: (617) 547-4648
       Schoenhof's Foreign Books: (617) 547-8855

🌐   harvard.com
       grolierpoetrybookshop.org
       schoenhofs.com

$ **Harvard Book Store:** Monday–Saturday, 9 a.m.–11p.m.; Sunday, 10 a.m.–10 p.m.
       Grolier Poetry Book Shop: Tuesday–Wednesday, 11 a.m.–7 p.m.;
       Thursday–Saturday, 11 a.m.–6 p.m.
       Schoenhof's Foreign Books: Monday–Friday, 10 a.m.–8 p.m.; Saturday, 10 a.m.–6 p.m.

🕐   Free, except for purchases

🚌   **T:** Red Line to Harvard Square

peaceful place 51

HATCH SHELL CONCERTS

Back Bay, Boston (MAP ONE)

CATEGORY ⌣ urban surprises ✪

*I*t used to be the locals' best-kept secret: the perfect time to catch the Fourth of July concert at the Hatch Shell was at the dress rehearsal on July 3. Now that people start lining up for that event at 6:30 in the morning, what's a music lover in search of serenity under the stars to do?

Fortunately, we have the Landmarks Orchestra. Every Wednesday night, mid-July–early September, this remarkable orchestra plays a free concert at the Hatch Shell. The concerts attract a diverse crowd: young people, baby boomer–aged couples, coworkers,

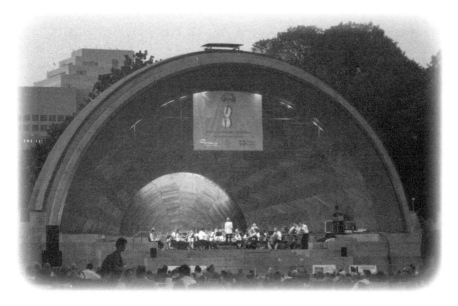

An enchanting evening at the Hatch Shell

families with children, and others in the know. It's common to arrive early, spread out a blanket, and relax with a picnic supper. (Leave the chilled rosé at home, though, as alcohol is not permitted on the Esplanade.) Should you wish something more comfortable than a blanket on which to rest, you can rent a chair for $5 or, of course, bring your own for free.

For those who prefer a little more solitude, come early and grab a bench facing the Charles River. You'll enjoy your own version of water music, watching the kayaks and sailboats float by as twilight settles over the river. A word to the wise: For true peacefulness, bring bug spray.

essentials

▣	Hatch Shell, Charles River Esplanade, 1 David G. Mugar Way, Boston, MA 02114
☎	**Landmarks Orchestra:** (617) 987-2000; **Hatch Shell:** (617) 626-4970
🌐	landmarksorchestra.org mass.gov/dcr/hatch_events.htm
$	Free
🕐	**Mid-July–early September:** Wednesday, 7 p.m.
🚍	**T:** Green Line, any train, to Arlington; Red Line to Charles/MGH. If walking isn't an option and you live too far from public transportation to this site, parking is allowed on the westbound lane of Storrow Drive on concert nights.

peaceful place 52

HEMLOCK GORGE RESERVATION

Newton Upper Falls and Needham, MA (MAP EIGHT)

CATEGORY ↙ outdoor habitats ✪ ✪ ✪

espite its location near the busy intersection of MA 9 and I-95, the primary sound at Hemlock Gorge is that of the Charles River pouring through the spillway that takes it under an old stone bridge as it rushes along on its journey to Boston. From this tranquil spot, you can walk the trails along the steep banks above the gorge, look for spotted sandpipers and other birdlife, or simply find a comfortable rock on which to picnic or savor a shady respite on a warm day. (Sadly, the hemlocks that give the gorge its name seem to be afflicted by the woolly adelgid pest that is devastating the hemlock population throughout the Northeast.)

Spanning the gorge is Echo Bridge, which is on the National Register of Historic Places and was once part of the aqueduct system that carried water into Boston. It's said that at the time the bridge was built, in 1877, it was the second-largest masonry arch in the United States. Children—as well as many adults—enjoy standing on the platform under the arch and sending their voices echoing throughout the gorge.

If you climb the stairs leading to the top of the bridge, you will be rewarded with fine treetop views of the river and surrounding area, including the falls that give Newton Upper Falls its name. The pathway is part of the Sudbury Aqueduct Linear District, a 16-mile historic area that goes from Framingham to the Chestnut Hill Reservoir. While I've never taken it, it's said to be an excellent hiking and biking path, with only a few minor interruptions.

↙ essentials

Bounded by Ellis Street and MA 9 in Newton Upper Falls, MA 02464, and Hamilton Place and Central Avenue in Needham, MA 02494

(C)   (617) 333-7404

(globe)   hemlockgorge.org; mass.gov/dcr/parks/metroboston/hemlock.htm

$ Free   (clock)   Daily, sunrise–sunset   (bus)   T: Green Line, D train, to Eliot

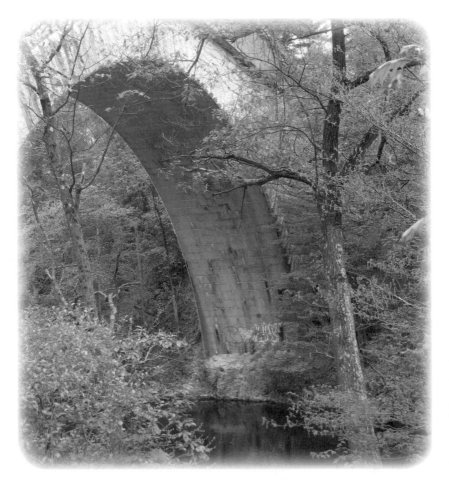

The arch at Echo Bridge

peaceful place 53

HONAN-ALLSTON BRANCH LIBRARY

Allston, Boston (MAPS FIVE AND SIX)

CATEGORY ↶ reading rooms ✪

*A*t most branch libraries, the books, CDs, or DVDs are the attractions. At the Honan-Allston branch, which opened in 2001, the library itself is the draw. With its alternating glass-walled reading rooms, courtyard reading gardens, and art gallery featuring works by local artists, the library offers a pleasant oasis in an otherwise busy corner of the city.

When the weather cooperates, the gardens tucked inside the 57,000-square-foot slate-, shingle-, and ironwood-clad building beckon you to come and escape into a good novel or just relax with your thoughts. On dreary days, the comfortable couches in the light-filled reading rooms facing the gardens are a perfect spot to curl up with a book or magazine.

One warning: Though there are designated adult's and children's sections, the building's open design means that when local schools bring their classes here for special events, the decibel level can climb more than a few notches above serenity. At those times, the park behind the library, with its shaded reading nook, winding paths, and enticing mist garden, can provide a tranquil alternative. Built on an abandoned industrial site as part of a collaborative effort among Harvard University, the city of Boston, and the Allston community, the 1.74-acre park has a man-made hilltop, where one can enjoy refreshing breezes and calming vistas.

↶ essentials

  300 North Harvard Street, Boston, MA 02134

ⓒ (617) 787-6313

🌐   bpl.org/branches/allston.htm   **$**   Free

🕐   Monday and Wednesday, noon–8 p.m.; Tuesday and Thursday, 10 a.m.–6 p.m.; Friday–Saturday, 9 a.m.–5 p.m.

🚌   **T:** Bus 66 (Harvard Square/Dudley Station via Allston and Brookline Village) to North Harvard Street

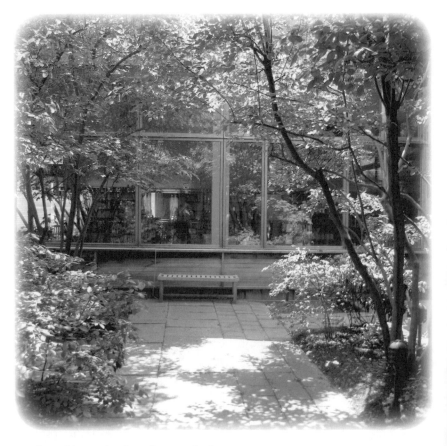

A peaceful atmosphere for reading or ruminating

peaceful place 54

HOUGHTON GARDEN

Chestnut Hill, MA (MAP EIGHT)

CATEGORY ⌣: parks & gardens ✪ ✪ ✪

In the spring, birdsong rings through the Houghton Garden as migrating warblers and thrushes seem to like to rest here on their journey north. And why not, because this little 10-acre wooded setting is a particularly alluring place. Begun by Martha Gilbert Houghton in 1906, it originally included an alpine rock garden; large stands of azaleas, rhododendrons, and exotic evergreens; a stream; and a lagoonlike pond. After decades

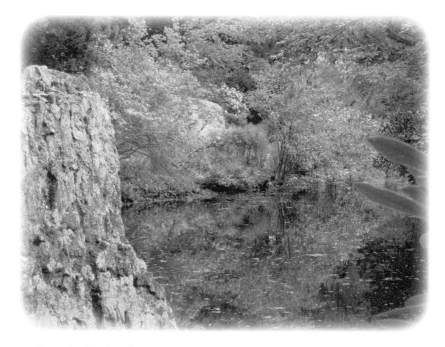

The pond at Houghton Garden

of neglect, the city of Newton rehabilitated the garden. Today, it's cared for under the auspices of the Chestnut Hill Garden Club.

In many ways, the Houghton Garden's current semiwild state seems to suit it. Beneath the trees at the Suffolk Road entrance, you'll see abundant clusters of naturalized lily of the valley; when in bloom, their enticing fragrance welcomes all who enter. The path around the pond is a lovely place to take a tranquil walk, with only the occasional sound of a passing Green Line train to remind you just how close to civilization you really are.

A brief ascent on stone steps brings you to the overlook, where a bench dedicated in Mrs. Houghton's memory provides a strategic resting spot with a view of the pond below. However, I find that the large puddingstone by the water's edge is a particularly inviting place to take a few moments to experience serenity and admire the vision that it took to create this special place, while acknowledging the impermanence of it all. Please note: In insect season, bug spray is a must.

∴ essentials

▱ Across from 162–210 Suffolk Road, Newton, MA 02467
If the gate at this location is locked, you can enter across the street from the Webster Conservation Area entrance, which is located around the corner from Suffolk Road.

☏ (617) 796-1134

☷ newtonconservators.org/19houghton.htm

$ Free

☼ Daily, sunrise–sunset

⛍ T: Green Line, D Train, to Chestnut Hill, then a 0.5-mile walk

peaceful place 55

HOWARD ULFELDER, MD, HEALING GARDEN

Beacon Hill, Boston (MAP TWO)

CATEGORY ⌣ scenic vistas ✪ ✪ ✪

The views of Beacon Hill, the Longfellow Bridge, and the Charles River from the secret terrace garden on the eighth floor of Massachusetts General Hospital's Yawkey Center for Outpatient Care are spectacular and inspiring. That's most appropriate because the Howard Ulfelder, MD, Healing Garden, which is located just down the corridor from the hospital's Cancer Center, was designed to provide both comfort and delight to those who are dealing with this dreaded illness: either a loved one's or their own.

Perhaps it's the sense of the life-and-death struggles going on around you here that makes this one of the most serene and contemplative places in Boston. The light-filled conservatory offers comfortable chairs and tropical plants. At the door that beckons you to the outdoors, a container of stones bears a sign welcoming you to take one.

Though the Healing Garden is small in size, it has been thoughtfully landscaped, with several areas in which to sit quietly and just be. I find that gazing into the poollike fountain, with its striking black square shape and bed of river stones, is particularly calming. Because the garden faces northwest, it's a magical place to watch the sunset over the Charles in those seasons when evening comes early. While the garden welcomes patients, visitors, and staff, on the occasions when I've been there, I've had the place to myself.

As you walk back to the elevator, be sure to read the inspiring stories told on the Cancer Center's Wall of Hope. You might be moved to whisper a prayer of good luck or blessing for those being treated here.

⌣ **essentials**

🖃 Eighth floor, Yawkey Center for Outpatient Care, 55 Fruit Street, Boston, MA 02114

📞 (617) 726-2000

massgeneral.org/services/outdoorspaces.aspx   **$**   Free

Monday–Friday, 9 a.m.–5 p.m.; closed holidays

T: Red Line to Charles/MGH

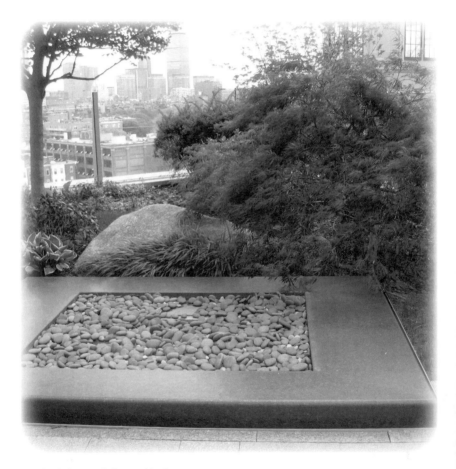

A calming spot for hope and healing

peaceful place 56

HUNGRY I

Beacon Hill, Boston (MAP TWO)

CATEGORY ⌣ quiet tables ✪

*R*estaurants can come and go quickly, so it says something that the Hungry I has been ensconced in a charming space in the basement of an 1840's Beacon Hill townhouse ever since the early 1980s. The food is French-bistro delicious, but it's the romantic atmosphere that makes the place so special: there's an authentic, woodburning fireplace in winter, a secluded backyard garden patio in summer, and three small rooms with antiques, paintings, and candlelit tables year-round.

The Hungry I is a very popular brunch and special-occasion dinner spot. So if you're looking for tranquility, I recommend lunch on Thursdays or Fridays. On cold winter days, you should request a fireside table. In summer, I'd recommend the garden patio—unless the weather is hot and humid. And I would imagine that the patio would also be a delightful place to drop into on a balmy evening for an appetizer and dessert under the stars—something I've promised myself that I will do in the near future.

⌣ essentials

▱ 71½ Charles Street, Boston, MA 02114

📞 (617) 227-3524   🌐 hungryiboston.com

$ **Lunch entrées:** $9–$19; **dinner entrées:** $25–$39; **brunch entrées:** $12–$24

🕐 Sunday–Wednesday, 5:30–9:30 p.m.; Thursday, noon–2 p.m. and 5:30–9:30 p.m.; Friday, noon–2 p.m. and 5:30–10 p.m.; Saturday, 5:30–10 p.m. **Brunch:** Sunday, 11 a.m.–2 p.m.

  T: Red Line to Charles/MGH

peaceful place 57

INN AT CASTLE HILL ON THE CRANE ESTATE

Ipswich, MA (MAP TEN)

CATEGORY ⌣ day trips & overnights ❂ ❂ ❂

*P*erhaps you're lucky enough to have friends who will invite you for a peaceful respite at their seaside country estate. If not, there's always the Inn at Castle Hill. Here, you can settle into a rocking chair on the wraparound porch and gaze across the tidal marsh to the ocean. Or curl up in the living room on a chilly evening and read by the fire. The inn, parts of which date from 1840, is one of the oldest structures on the Trustees of Reservations' Crane Estate, site of the magnificent 59-room Great House built in 1928.

Like those who come for the day, you can stroll about the estate's newly restored Italianate garden, savor dramatic views from the 0.5-mile-long Grand Allée, or take a tour of the mansion. If you'd like to meander on, there are paths through the woods and a trail that takes you past meadows and marshes to secluded Cedar Point and on to Steep Hill Beach. (On weekends, the estate can be quite popular, though the crowds seem to almost magically disappear by late afternoon.)

Inn guests are welcome to walk the dune path to the less-visited side of Crane Beach or to launch a kayak from the private dock and take a tranquil paddle through the Essex River estuary. If it's not beach weather, borrow a bicycle for a ride by the orchards and marshes along Argilla Road or explore the antiques shops that dot MA 133. (However, on warm, sunny days, traffic can make the bicycling or antiquing option anything but serene.)

The inn's 10 comfortably luxurious rooms offer woodland or marsh and ocean views. (If you're a sunrise enthusiast, the latter are worth the extra dollars.) Innkeepers serve a hearty breakfast in the sun-drenched morning room. At night, stars parade across the sky, and at all times you're never far from the salty smell of the sea.

Though 2-night stays are the rule on weekends—3 on holidays—it's often possible to arrange an overnight midweek. One caution: The greenhead flies that emerge from the marshes for a few weeks here in July can be fierce.

Note: The Castle Hill Inn in Newport, Rhode Island, is a Relais & Châteaux property, not to be confused with the Inn at Castle Hill in Massachusetts.

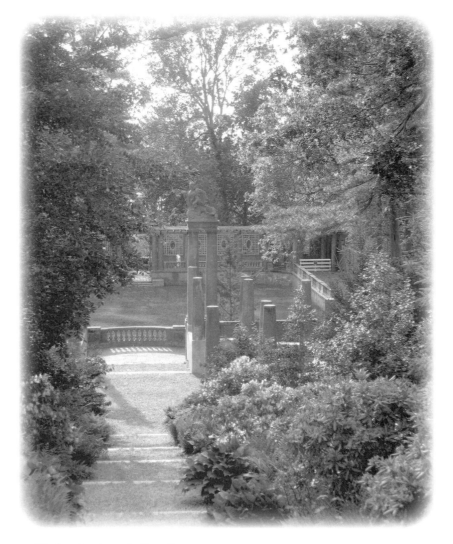

The formal gardens at the Crane Estate

⌣ essentials

 Inn: 280 Argilla Road; **Estate:** 290 Argilla Road, Ipswich, Massachusetts 01938

ℰ **Inn:** (978) 412-2555; **Estate:** (978) 356-4351

🌐 **Inn:** thetrustees.org/the-inn-at-castle-hill
Estate: thetrustees.org (Click on "Places to Visit," then "List of Reservations," and choose "Castle Hill at Crane Estate.")

$ **Inn:** April and November–December: $140–$350; May–October: $175–$385; closed January–March
Estate and grounds: Memorial Day weekend–Labor Day weekend: Saturday–Sunday and holiday Mondays: $8 per car; $5 per car all other times; $2 per bicycle year-round; $4 per motorcycle year-round; Ipswich residents: free, Monday–Friday, same admission fees as nonmembers Saturday–Sunday; Trustees members: free year-round. See website above for information on Great House and Historic Landscape tours.

🕐 **Inn:** April–December. **Estate and grounds:** Daily, 8 a.m.–sunset

🚗 n/a

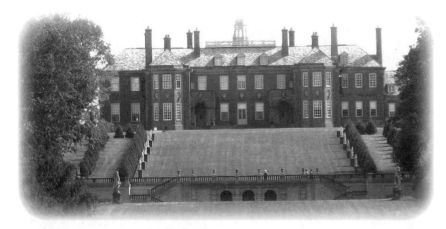

The estate's Great House as seen from the Grand Allée

peaceful place 58

THE INSTITUTE OF CONTEMPORARY ART, BOSTON

Fan Pier, Boston (MAP FOUR)

CATEGORY ⌣ museums & galleries ⭐

To me, The Institute of Contemporary Art (ICA), Boston, which juts out over the edge of Boston Harbor, looks like a diver up on her toes, preparing to leap. This little steel-and-glass jewel box of a museum occupies one of the most spectacular settings along the Boston HarborWalk. That makes this a splendid spot for admiring the views both inside and out.

The museum, which celebrates contemporary works in all media, from visual art to video, is slowly accumulating an impressive permanent collection. This art, plus special

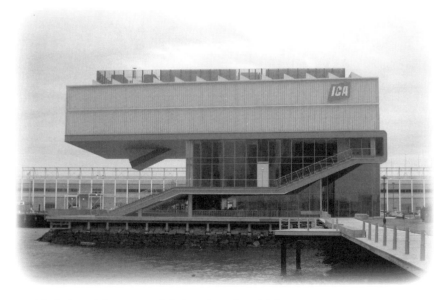

The Institute of Contemporary Art's dramatic cantilevered design

exhibits that change on a regular basis, are displayed on the museum's fourth floor. When you're ready to shift your gaze outward, head to the Founders Gallery, where you can usually find a space on one of the five padded benches that face the water. Here, through floor-to-ceiling windows that span the width of the museum, you can savor sky, city, and seascape dappled by nature's ever-changing hues. Or go one floor below, and curl up on the pillowed bleacherlike seating in the media center, where you'll have the sensation of floating above the waves, unanchored by either horizon or sky.

The Water Café on the ground floor is a pleasant place to enjoy a meal or a snack—and even more so after its fall 2011 post-renovation reopening. On nice days, the seating spills out onto an open-air deck. If you're in the mood for a stunning sunset, and the weather is cooperative, it's hard to imagine a more remarkable panorama than the one you'll see from the ICA's harbor-front plaza. Just sit back and get ready to enjoy the show.

✓ essentials

100 Northern Avenue, Boston, MA 02210

(617) 478-3100

icaboston.org

$ Adults: $15; seniors: $13; students: $10; children age 17 and younger and members: free; Thursday, 5–9 p.m.: free; last Saturday of each month (except December): free for families (up to two adults accompanied by children age 12 and younger)

Tuesday–Wednesday, 10 a.m.–5 p.m.; Thursday–Friday, 10 a.m.–9 p.m.; Saturday–Sunday, 10 a.m.–5 p.m.

T: Silver Line, Waterfront, to Courthouse or World Trade Center

peaceful place 59

ISABELLA STEWART GARDNER MUSEUM

The Fenway, Boston (MAP FIVE)

CATEGORY ⌣ museums & galleries ✪

*I*sabella Stewart Gardner created quite a scandal when she abandoned her Back Bay townhouse for a mansion in a marshy area of the Fenway. Today, the place she called Fenway Court is one of Boston's most beloved museums.

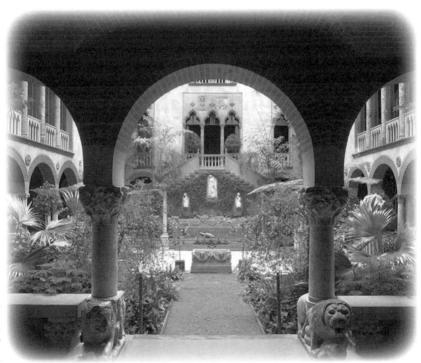

photographed by Clements/Howcroft 2008

"Mrs. Jack's" creation

Inspired by a 15th-century Venetian palazzo, the building is centered around a glass-covered courtyard, where nine spectacular, themed floral garden displays are rotated with the seasons. (If the profusion of orchids and bromeliads in late winter don't chase away your blues, nothing will.)

Mrs. Jack, as she was called, was a voracious collector, so art is everywhere you look—from the architectural elements and textiles to furniture and decorative objects to sculpture, rare books, and paintings. According to the museum's website, this is the only private art collection in which the building and collection are the creation of one individual.

Among the many masterpieces are works by Rembrandt van Rijn, Michelangelo Buonarroti, Sandro Botticelli, and Edgar Degas. One of my favorite paintings, John Singer Sargent's evocative *El Jaleo,* has a prominent spot near the courtyard. My other favorite, *The Concert* by Johannes Vermeer, is sadly missing, as it was stolen during the infamous March 1990 art heist.

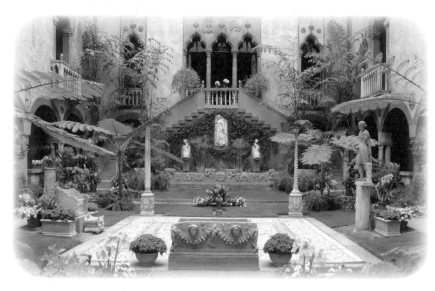

The interior central courtyard in bloom

photographed by Thomas Lingner 2008

The museum's intimate scale is one of its great appeals, though it makes avoiding the crowds on weekends a bit of a challenge. My suggestion? Try to arrive just at the 11 a.m. opening. Another idea: I find the most magical time to visit is during one of the Gardner After Hours events, held 5:30–9:30 p.m. on the third Thursday of every month. Come early so you have plenty of time to listen to music while you relax along the cloister wall with a glass of wine. Then explore the upstairs galleries. You're welcome to stop and sketch in the Dutch Room; pencil and paper are even provided.

On those evenings, I especially enjoy lingering at the windows and admiring the way the courtyard and cloisters look when lit by sconce light. It makes me feel that I've been transported back in time to one of Mrs. Jack's soirées.

Note: After a respite during 2011, Gardner After Hours events resume in February 2012 following the opening of the Renzo Piano–designed wing.

essentials

🖅 280 The Fenway, Boston, MA 02115

📞 **Information:** (617) 566-1401; **Box office:** (617) 278-5156

🌐 gardnermuseum.org

$ **Adults:** $12; **seniors:** $10; **college students with current ID:** $5; **children age 17 and younger, those named Isabella, and members:** free

🕐 Tuesday–Sunday, 11 a.m.–5 p.m.; closed July 4, Thanksgiving, and December 25

🚌 **T:** Green Line, E train, to Museum of Fine Arts

peaceful place 60

JAMAICA POND

Jamaica Plain, Boston (MAP EIGHT)

CATEGORY ↲ outdoor habitats ⊛

*J*amaica Pond can be a boisterous place. When the weather cooperates, the 1.5-mile path around the perimeter is full of walkers, joggers, kids, dogs, and, here and there, even a fisherman with a line out for trout or salmon.

But when the path is lively, the pond itself beckons. Though it was once a source of water for residents of Boston—and for their ice in winter—today, the spring-fed pond serves as a refuge in the heart of the city. In season, you may rent kayaks, rowboats, and sailboats* by the hour at the picturesque Tudor-inspired boathouse. While a kayak is perfect for solitary exploration in the pond, a rowboat enables you to share the experience with family or friends. Bring a picnic and, if you want to exercise your artistry, a sketchbook: the pond offers lovely views of the surrounding Jamaica Pond Park and beyond.

For a particularly magical experience, don't miss the Lantern Parade in late October. Plan to arrive just before sunset when the hushed crowd sets out to circle the pond carrying candlelit lanterns handmade from recycled soda bottles and colored tissue paper. (The boathouse hosts lantern-making workshops in the fall, or you can purchase one the night of the parade.) It's hard to decide which is more delightful—joining in the parade or contemplating the magical spectacle of sparkling light from a distance.

*Note: Sailboats are not available when the Summer Youth Program is in session. Private boats are not allowed.

↲ essentials

| ≡ | **Boathouse:** 507 Jamaica Way, Jamaica Plain, MA 02130 |

| *C* | **Boathouse:** May–November 2: (617) 522-5061; November 3–April: (617) 242-3821, ext. 12 |

🌐 jamaicapond.com
emeraldnecklace.org/the-parks

$ **Rentals (per hour):** Rowboats: $10 ($5 with fishing license); kayaks: $12; sailboats: $15

🕐 **Jamaica Pond Park:** Daily, 6 a.m.–11:30 p.m. **Boathouse:** May–November 2: Daily, 11 a.m.–7 p.m.

🚇 **T:** Orange Line to Green Street; Bus 39 (Forest Hills/Back Bay Station via Huntington Avenue) to Centre Street

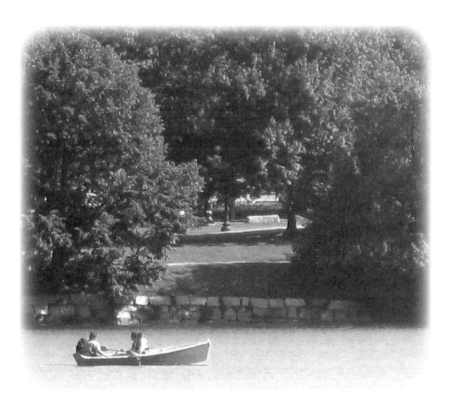

Boating on Jamaica Pond

peaceful place 61

JOHN F. KENNEDY MEMORIAL PARK

Cambridge, MA (MAP SIX)

CATEGORY ↙ parks & gardens ⭐

*I*t was John F. Kennedy's cherished dream that his presidential library would occupy a site overlooking the Charles River, next to Harvard University. However, his aspiration faced years of opposition from community activists concerned about the deleterious effects of increased traffic in already busy Harvard Square. So, the library ultimately was built in Dorchester on a point of land that juts out into Boston Harbor. And

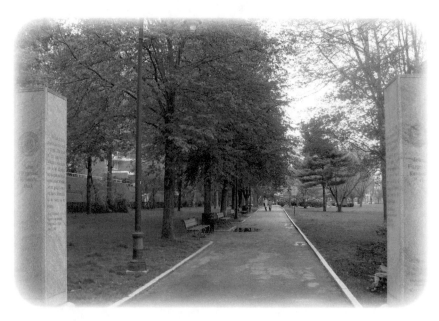

The entrance to John F. Kennedy Memorial Park

instead, the place called "the closest to his [JFK's] heart" became the commonwealth's official memorial to the 35th president.

When you walk down the tranquil landscaped passageway from Eliot Street through the entrance pillars to the park that bears his name, it's easy to see why President Kennedy was so fond of this spot. This is the quiet, sycamore-lined stretch of Memorial Drive. There is a huge expanse of shade-dappled lawn where you can stretch out and watch the sculls go racing down the Charles.

The memorial is centered on a large fountain. When it's working, all you hear is the sound of water and perhaps the wind in the trees. Though the riverbank across the way is always busy with joggers, in-line skaters, and bicyclists, the park exudes an air of serenity. Except on balmy Sundays, I've never seen more than a few people here at any one time.

The plantings, mostly natives, bloom in May, the late president's birthday month, which makes that the ideal time to visit.

↩ essentials

✉	970 Memorial Drive, Cambridge, MA 02138
☎	n/a
🌐	n/a
$	Free
🕐	Daily, sunrise–sunset
🚇	**T:** Red Line to Harvard Square

peaceful place 62

JOHN JOSEPH MOAKLEY U.S. COURTHOUSE

Fan Pier, Boston (MAP FOUR)

CATEGORY ✧ urban surprises ✪

*I*t may seem a bit unusual to recommend a courthouse as a destination for anyone other than an attorney, juror, or defendant, let alone for someone in search of scenery and serenity. But the Moakley Courthouse (in shorthand) is more than a place of justice. This singular waterfront edifice was designed by Henry Cobb, the architect responsible for the John Hancock building in the Back Bay. Like that building, the Moakley Courthouse makes a striking visual statement; in this case it's with an 88-foot-high curved glass wall that, from inside the building, delivers a sweeping panorama of sky, harbor, and city.

As much as I love the inspiring scenery outside, I find myself drawn to the 10-story-high rotunda in the heart of the building. There, on circular walls, you'll see 9 of minimalist artist Ellsworth Kelly's 21 fiberglass-and-aluminum *Boston Panels*, each a single, brilliant color. Looking up at those 11-by-13^1/$_2$-foot panels, I find myself transfixed by their vivid patches of horizontal color, illuminated by light streaming down through the rotunda's skylight. (The remaining 12 panels, measuring 11 feet by 88 inches, frame each side of the great window on six floors of the building. You can catch glimpses of them from the rotunda.)

If abstract art isn't your thing, you may want to wander through the Moakley's public gallery spaces, where the exhibits change on a regular basis. You're also welcome to visit the ninth-floor law library, which offers a quiet space to read and take in expansive views of Fan Pier and Fort Point Channel.

Should you desire a place to linger, there's a small café (open until 2:30 p.m.) on the second floor where you can grab a window-side table and admire the vista in relative peace; unless it's lunchtime, you will likely be alone with your thoughts.

In winter, when dusk comes before closing time at the Moakley, the great window offers dramatic views of colors playing on the waters of the inner harbor as the sun sets behind the city. If it's a clear evening, walk across the channel via the Northern Avenue Bridge and turn around to admire the sight of the Kelly panels shining like oversize gems through the courthouse windows.

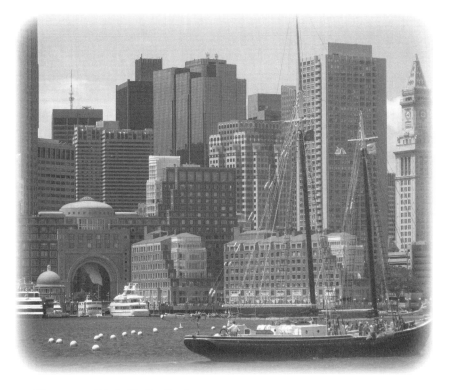

The scenery outside the Moakley Courthouse

⌣ essentials

☞ 1 Courthouse Way, Boston, MA 02210

✆ (617) 261-2440

🌐 moakleycourthouse.com

$ n/a

🕐 Monday–Friday, 8:30 a.m.–5 p.m.; closed all federal holidays.
    Café: Monday–Friday, 9 a.m.–2:30 p.m.

🚌 **T:** Red Line to South Station

peaceful place 63

JORDAN HALL, NEW ENGLAND CONSERVATORY

The Fenway, Boston (MAP FIVE)

CATEGORY urban surprises ✪ ✪

Symphony Hall is rightly considered a Boston treasure, but little more than two blocks away, you'll find another exquisite setting for concerts: the New England Conservatory's Jordan Hall. High praise abounds for this site and tends to focus on the structure's acoustic perfection.

Intimate in scale, Jordan Hall—which opened in 1903 and earned National Historic Landmark status 91 years later—was inspired by the concert halls that Renaissance

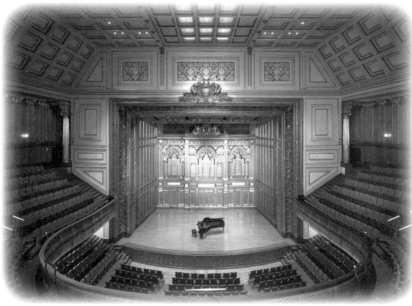

The view from the balcony at Jordan Hall

photographed by Nick Wheeler

nobles built for their courts. I find Jordan Hall to be both lovely and a bit quirky; in the balcony, the rows of seats tilt noticeably stage-ward, while on the main floor, certain seats seem to randomly block aisles. But nowhere else do you feel as close to the music and musicians. And what music there is!

On any given evening, September–May, you can wander into Jordan Hall and be entranced by anything from jazz to string quartets to opera—performed by students, faculty, distinguished alumni, or outside guests. Not only are most of the concerts free, but you're also welcome to sit wherever you please. While the First Monday at Jordan Hall concert series is usually well attended, at other performances, you may feel as though the musicians are playing especially for you. Recitals and master classes held in other performance spaces throughout the conservatory's campus are also open to the public.

⌣ essentials

✉   30 Gainesborough Street, Boston, MA 02115

☎   (617) 585-1260

🌐   necmusic.edu/jordan-hall

$ Most concerts are free; check with box office.

🕐   **Box office:** Monday–Friday, 10 a.m.–6 p.m.; Saturday, noon–6 p.m. Check with box office for specific performance times.

🚇   **T:** Green Line, E train, to Symphony

peaceful place 64

JUDSON B. COIT OBSERVATORY, BOSTON UNIVERSITY

Kenmore Square, Boston (MAP FIVE)

CATEGORY ∴ urban surprises ✪

A suggestion: Some Wednesday evening, take the elevator to the fifth floor at 725 Commonwealth and walk down the hallway to the first open door. Climb one flight of stairs, and then follow the red lights out to the roof. You've just discovered one of the least-known nighttime vantage points in the city: the observatory at Boston University. Ostensibly, you're here for one of the astronomy department's Public Open Nights, where you can see the heavens through the observatory's 8-inch telescopes. But

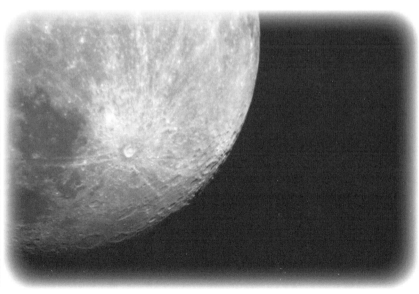

A telescopic view of the moon

you'll also experience one of the most spectacular yet tranquil after-dark vistas in the city. From here, panoramic views sweep up to and across the Charles River, to Cambridge, and to downtown Boston.

Of course, for the observatory to hold Public Open Nights, the skies must be clear. That is not an easy feat in the city, especially in springtime or on hazy, humid summer nights. On winter nights, when cloudless skies are more common, the cold presents its own challenges for outdoor stargazers, so dress accordingly. Fortunately, the observatory has a call line (see "essentials," below), which broadcasts the go/no-go decision about 2 hours ahead of time. (You can also get updates via Twitter: @buobservatory.)

On optimum sky-viewing nights, the event can attract a good number of students and local astronomy buffs. Still there's usually a hushed, unhurried atmosphere up here, and the lines for the telescopes move quite quickly. Whenever I do this, I like to bring along binoculars so I can scan both heaven and earth while waiting my turn at the telescopes.

essentials

725 Commonwealth Avenue, Boston, MA 02215

(617) 353-2630

bu.edu/astronomy/events/public-open-night-at-the-observatory
bu.edu/astronomy/astronomy-department-facilities/judson-b-coit-observatory

$ Free

Spring–summer: Wednesday, 8:30–9:30 p.m. **Fall–winter:** Wednesday, 7:30–8:30 p.m.

T: Green Line, B train, to Boston University East

peaceful place 65

KAJI ASO STUDIO INSTITUTE FOR THE ARTS

The Fenway, Boston (MAP FIVE)

CATEGORY ⌣ spiritual enclaves ✪ ✪ ✪

chi go ichi e: "one meeting, full of friendship." That's the motto of the special tea ceremonies held every Sunday at the Kaji Aso Studio Institute for the Arts, just down the street from Symphony Hall. But it also applies to most of the activities that take place in this tranquil brownstone that is an art school, gallery, concert hall, teahouse, and garden—all in one location.

The institute's namesake, Kaji Aso, was an artist, calligrapher, poet, and professor, first at Tufts University and later at the School of the Museum of Fine Arts, in Boston. He was also a master of the Japanese tea ceremony. Kate Finnegan, who apprenticed with Aso from 1980 until his death in 2006, now carries on the tradition. Limited to six

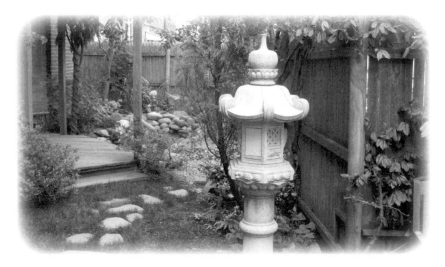

On the way to the teahouse

participants, the weekly ceremony unfolds in a secluded teahouse. To get there, you pass through an intricately landscaped garden, complete with perennials, flowering fruit trees, water features, and a small yet exquisite fishpond.

The teahouse, with its tatami-mat floors, is a relaxed place where time seems to stand still, yet flows with the seasons. The main elements of the ceremony—the art on the walls, the kimonos worn by the hostess, and the choice of tea bowls and pastries—all change as the year unfolds. The tranquil, meditative atmosphere—where the rich aromas of grassy green tea, incense, and burning hardwood mingle—seems to create a special bond among participants, even those who began the ceremony as strangers.

The institute also offers a regular schedule of events as well as classes in painting, ceramics, philosophy, music, poetry, and Japanese culture. Some of the classes are even welcome to drop-ins, if you feel so inspired, though advance notice is always appreciated.

In the Boston Public Garden, there's a Japanese mountain cherry tree dedicated to Kaji Aso. Appropriately, there's a plaque bearing one of his nontraditional haiku:

End of day
still,
cherry petals are flying
To which I can only reply: "Ah, yes, they are!"

✧ essentials

✉	40 St. Stephen Street, Boston, MA 02115	☎	(617) 247-1719

🌐 kajiasostudio.com $ **Gallery:** free. **Tea ceremony:** $30

🕐 **Gallery:** Tuesday, 1–9 p.m.; Wednesday–Friday, 1–5 p.m.; Saturday, 2–4 p.m., or by appointment. **Tea ceremony:** Sunday, 4–6 p.m.; reservations required

🚇 **T:** Green Line, E train, to Symphony

peaceful place 66

KELLEHER ROSE GARDEN

The Fenway, Boston (MAP FIVE)

CATEGORY ⌣ parks & gardens ✪ ✪

*I*magine a secluded garden where 1,500 roses of nearly 200 varieties—from shrub roses to climbers, floribundas to hybrid teas, and grandifloras to David Austins—are all in bloom at the same time! That's what you'll find when you venture to the Kelleher Rose Garden in late spring.

Noted landscape architect Arthur Shurcliff designed the original circular garden with its grand central fountain in 1931. (A protégé of Frederick Law Olmsted, who created Boston's Emerald Necklace system of parks, Shurcliff was responsible for designing the

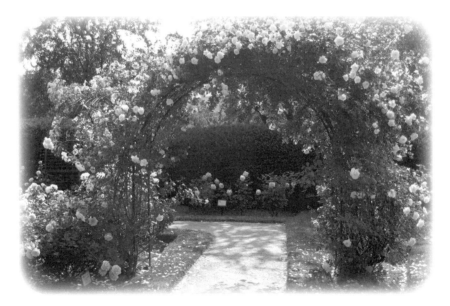

The rose garden in June

Charles River Esplanade, as well as for the restoration of the impressive Colonial gardens in Williamsburg, Virginia.)

In its early days, the rose garden was such a popular place for Bostonians to promenade that the rectangular section—with its gently curving paths, rose-covered arbors, and shady seating nooks—was added just a few years later. By the end of the 20th century, however, a long period of neglect and decline had taken its toll. Happily, after an 8-year restoration by the Emerald Necklace Conservancy and the Boston Parks & Recreation department, the garden once again provides an intoxicating kaleidoscope of fragrance and color. (It's anticipated that soon, the sound of the restored fountain will add to the sensory symphony.)

At peak blooming season, the garden is a favored spot for garden club tours and weddings. So I find that early mornings, when the blossoms are still dew-drenched, are an especially enticing time to visit. Fragrance is most alluring on warm afternoons, when the garden becomes a tempting place to sit with a book or watercolors. On Tuesday evenings spring–fall, volunteers gather 5:30–7:30 p.m. to prune and deadhead the roses; thanks to their loving care, there will be blossoms here to delight you all season long.

essentials

⊡   Agassiz Road and Park Drive, Boston, MA 02215

📞   (617) 522-2700

🌐   emeraldnecklace.org (Type "Kelleher Rose Garden" into the search box.)

$ Free

🕐   **May–mid-November:** Daily, sunrise–sunset

🚌   **T:** Green Line, E train, to Museum of Fine Arts

peaceful place 67

KEVIN W. FITZGERALD PARK
Mission Hill, Boston (MAP EIGHT)
CATEGORY scenic vistas ⭐

rban serenity seekers in need of a quiet spot with cool breezes and inspiring vistas would be wise to venture up St. Alphonsus Street to the 5.5-acre Kevin W. Fitzgerald Park, near the top of Mission Hill. Here, one can gaze out over the twin spires of the Basilica of Our Lady of Perpetual Help—the mission church that gave the hill its name—and enjoy a magnificent panorama of Brookline, the Back Bay, and downtown Boston. The basilica's bells, which ring every quarter hour, as proper church bells should, augment the rather pastoral surroundings.

The park, with its winding paths, manicured lawns, and meadowlike wilds scattered

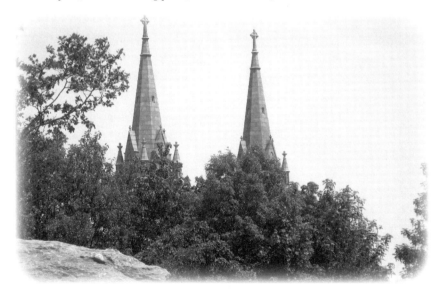

A hilltop view toward the twin spires of the Basilica of Our Lady of Perpetual Help

with poppies and lupine, was originally named Puddingstone Park after the stone that was once quarried here. (In fact, it makes up the bedrock layer on which Roxbury and numerous neighboring towns sit.) This fascinating stone remains much in evidence at Kevin W. Fitzgerald: pillars of puddingstone support the steel archway that welcomes visitors at the park's entrance; walls of the circa 1843 quarry form the backdrop for the serpentine path that leads back down to Tremont Street; and strategically placed boulders serve as delightful places to perch and admire the view.

So what exactly is puddingstone? Numerous markers throughout the park tell the tale of this far-from-humble sedimentary deposit that's theorized to contain layers between 570 million and 600 million years old. To me, the highlight is poet Oliver Wendell Holmes's homage from his 1859 essay *The Professor at the Breakfast-Table*: ". . . a lump of puddingstone is a thing to look at, to think about, to study over, to dream upon, to go crazy with . . . Look at that pebble in it. From what cliff was it broken? On what beach rolled by the waves of what ocean? How and when embedded in soft ooze, which itself became stone, and by-and-by was lifted onto bald summits and steep cliffs?" The basilica itself, below the hilltop park, is built from Roxbury puddingstone, possibly even rock quarried from this very spot.

The park is closed when snow and ice are present, which is a wise thing, as the thought of sledding here is as tempting as it would be foolhardy. While I've usually found that this spot is quite serene, should you find it too crowded for your tastes or should you wish a less strenuous climb, the basilica's garden also offers a splendid view of the surroundings.

↙ essentials

⌗   174 St. Alphonsus Street, Boston, MA 02120

☎   (617) 566-6565   ⚑   missionhillnhs.org/puddingstone-park

$ Free

🕐   **Memorial Day weekend–September:** Daily, 6 a.m.–9 p.m. **October–late May:** Daily, 6 a.m.–sunset; closed for snow and ice

🚈   **T:** Green Line, E train, to Brigham Circle; Orange Line to Roxbury Crossing

peaceful place 68

LALA ROKH

Beacon Hill, Boston (MAP TWO)

CATEGORY ↵ quiet tables ✪ ✪

*F*rom the moment you walk through the door at 97 Mount Vernon Street, you feel genuinely welcomed, as though you've been invited into someone's home. In this case, that sentiment is not misplaced. Lala Rokh is owned by a brother and sister; many of the dishes served here are based on recipes their mother brought with her when she left Azerbaijan in northwestern Iran, and the decor even incorporates some of the family's collection of 16th-century and 17th-century Persian miniatures. (The name Lala Rokh means "tulip cheeks" in Persian and comes from a 19th-century English epic romance celebrating the mysteries of the East.)

Lala Rokh defies the current—and somewhat annoying—restaurant trend of loud music and tables crowded together. Instead, a cozy bar sits off to the left as you enter, and the pale yellow walls in the main dining rooms create a warm and inviting atmosphere. It's a quiet place to linger over a romantic dinner à deux or to relax with friends and enjoy a conversation. It's also a wonderful getaway for a tranquil solo lunch; you can read a book or write in your journal while you savor unusual, aromatic dishes seasoned with exotic spices and herbs.

↵ essentials

✉ 97 Mount Vernon Street, Boston, MA 02108   ☏ (617) 720-5511

🌐 lalarokh.com $ **Appetizers:** $5–$8; **entrées:** $14–$19

🕐 Monday–Friday, noon-2 p.m. and 5:30–10 p.m.; Saturday–Sunday, 5:30–10 p.m.

🚆 **T:** Red Line to Charles/MGH; Green Line, any train, to Arlington or Boylston

peaceful place 69

LANNAN SHIP MODEL GALLERY

Waterfront District, Boston (MAP THREE)

CATEGORY ⌣ shops & services ✪ ✪

*L*ong before Boston became a mecca for high tech, biotech, and mutual funds, the city was a hub of maritime activity. The Lannan Ship Model Gallery offers a fascinating glimpse into those times. This 6,000-square-foot store is said to be the largest marine gallery in the world.

A treasure trove of marine paintings and antique charts—along with rare lithographs, photographs, and engravings—await your viewing. You'll also find a complete array of

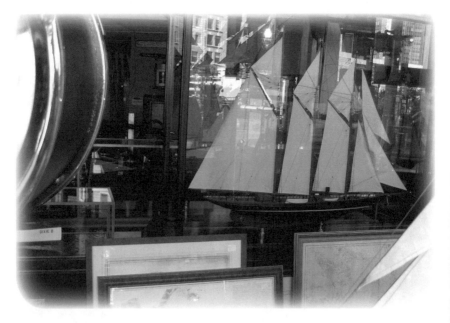

A hint of the treasures inside

nautical memorabilia, from foghorns and sea chests to ships' bells and block and tackle deadeyes. Need a nautical-themed sign or some bric-a-brac for your Cape house? This is the place to look. However, most items are antiques and are priced accordingly.

As its name implies, the store features a breathtaking collection of ship's models, its true claim to fame. More than 40 models on display at any one time will surely capture your attention, and the collection usually includes a fully rigged replica of the USS *Constitution*. You'll even find vintage pond yachts ready to sail on the Charles River Esplanade or Jamaica Pond. And the staff takes a true delight in their offerings. While they welcome browsers, they're more than happy to spend time pointing out the highlights of the Lannan Gallery in intricate detail.

essentials

🖃   99 High Street, Boston, MA 02110

☎   (617) 451-2650

🌐   lannangallery.com

$ Free, except for purchases

🕓   Monday–Friday, 10:30 a.m.–4 p.m.; Saturday, 12:30 p.m.–4 p.m.; also by appointment

🚇   **T:** Red Line to South Station

peaceful place 70

LECHMERE CANAL PARK

East Cambridge, MA (MAP SEVEN)

CATEGORY ⌣ parks & gardens ✪ ✪

*T*he 7.5-acre Lechmere Canal Park was built to provide a link between the East Cambridge community and the Charles River. Despite its proximity to the CambridgeSide Galleria, I find that it is a lovely escape from the crowds of bicyclists, joggers, and walkers that often crowd the banks of the Charles.

It's hard to believe that, not too long ago, this vibrant neighborhood—which now offers myriad places to live, shop, work, and relax—was once a blighted industrial zone. (The placid canal is built on the site of an industrial waterway that was used to bring raw

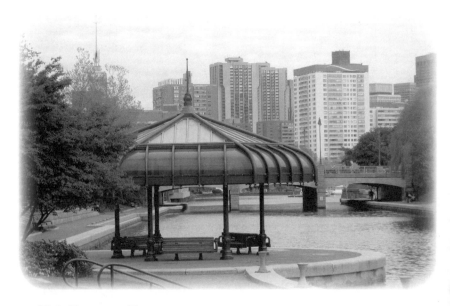

The inviting water pavilion

materials into the area's factories and deliver the finished products to nearby rail yards.) The spectacular public fountain, said to be New England's tallest, not only provides a dramatic focal point, but it also serves to muffle the traffic noises from nearby Edwin H. Land Boulevard and Monsignor O'Brien Highway. Though I've never seen anyone use it, a stepped granite seawall enables those with small boats to easily exit the park and enter the water. Benches both at the water's edge and in the lushly landscaped areas of the park provide places to rest and enjoy the cool river breezes.

The charming water pavilion, which was designed to serve as a theater stage and band shell, as well as a comfortable place to pause and enjoy the surroundings, displays a brief history of the area, complete with vintage photographs etched into the glass panels.

✌ essentials

📧 Off Cambridge Parkway, between Edwin H. Land Boulevard and Monsignor O'Brien Parkway, Cambridge, MA 02141

📞 n/a

🌐 n/a

$ Free

🕐 Open 24/7

🚆 **T:** Green Line, Lechmere train, to Science Park

peaceful place 71

LEWIS WHARF HIDDEN GARDEN

Wharf District, Boston (MAP THREE)

CATEGORY ⌣ urban surprises ✪ ✪ ✪

*I*t's a rare garden that offers year-round charm, but this little-known jewel, the Lewis Wharf Hidden Garden, is such a place. Designed by Carl Koch in the early 1970s in memory of his wife, Ruth Chamberlain Koch, this secret haven nestles between Commercial Street and the harbor, beside the Lewis Wharf condominiums.

I particularly love the rear section, which echoes the style of an 18th-century pleasure garden, with geometric boxwood-edged beds set out along a winding gravel path. Here under huge yew hedges, two small benches face each other. It's a cozy spot, protected

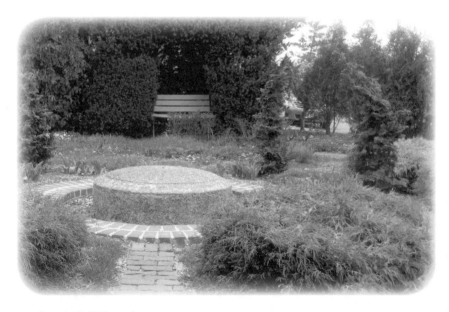

A seat in the hidden garden

from the wind. On foggy or snowy days in early winter, before the resident robins and mockingbirds have stripped the bright red fruit from the nearby crab apple trees, it's absolutely magical here.

On weekends, in warmer seasons, the grassy area near the front provides a tempting space for families to picnic while the kids frolic on the lawn. An herb garden and rose beds perfume the air, accompanied by the sound of a small fountain. By late afternoon, a sense of calm settles in, which makes that the perfect time to sit on a bench and share a quiet conversation or simply enjoy a refreshing sea breeze.

⌣ essentials

✉	Off Commercial Street at Lewis Wharf, Boston, MA 02110
✆	(617) 482-1722
⊕	bostonharborwalk.com/placestogo
$	Free
⊙	Daily, sunrise–sunset
🚋	**T:** Blue Line to Aquarium; Orange Line or Green Line, any train, to Haymarket

peaceful place 72

LONGFELLOW HOUSE GARDENS

Cambridge, MA (MAP SIX)

CATEGORY ↙ parks & gardens ✪ ✪ ✪

*N*o matter how many times I pass this block of Brattle Street, I always
feel a slight sense of surprise as the large yellow Colonial-era mansion emerges,
with its big trees and wide lawns that extend all the way to Mount Auburn Street and
vistas that stretch beyond to the banks of the Charles.

"I wonder who lived here," I thought the first time I saw it. The answer is as illustrious
as the setting: during the Siege of Boston, July 1775–April 1776, the house was headquarters for General George Washington. Poet Henry Wadsworth Longfellow also lived

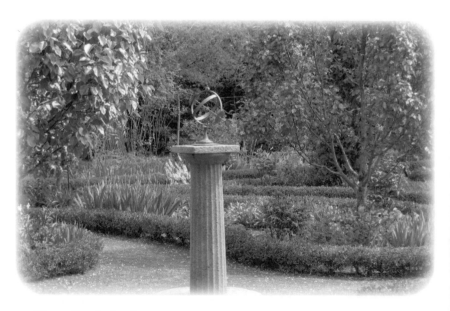

The recently restored garden

there from 1837 until his death in 1882. (While he started his life there as a boarder, his father-in-law gave him the house as a wedding present in 1843.)

Today, the mansion is a historic site managed by the National Park Service. While tours of the house are given only in summer, you may enjoy the grounds and the formal garden year-round. And what a magnificent garden it is! Located far enough back from busy Brattle Street to be sheltered from noise, the tranquil space offers a haven of sensory pleasure. On sunny Sundays in spring, one feels incomparably serene, sitting in the shade of the pergola; inhaling the scent of lilacs, blossoming ornamental fruit trees, or roses; and listening to the church bells of Cambridge ring in the distance. A restoration completed in 2006 re-created the garden's original design and palette, adding 1,700 tiny Korean boxwoods to replicate the low hedges that Longfellow himself had laid out.

Alas, the large canopied tree on the side lawn is a linden, not the spreading chestnut celebrated in Longfellow's famous poem about the village blacksmith. Apparently, when that tree had to be cut down, local schoolchildren raised money so that some of the wood could be made into a chair that was then given to the poet; today that chair still sits in Longfellow's study.

⌣ essentials

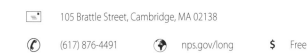

📧 105 Brattle Street, Cambridge, MA 02138

☎ (617) 876-4491   🌐 nps.gov/long $ Free

🕐 **Gardens and grounds:** Daily, sunrise–sunset. **House:** June–October: Wednesday–Sunday, tours at 10:30 a.m., 11:30 a.m., 1 p.m., 2 p.m., 3 p.m., and 4 p.m. (In July–August, the last Sunday tour is at 3 p.m.)

🚇 **T:** Red Line to Harvard

peaceful place 73

LYMAN ESTATE GREENHOUSES
Waltham, MA (MAP NINE)
CATEGORY ↙ historic sites ✪ ✪

y mid-February, the grayest, dreariest part of winter has usually settled into the Boston area, leaving most of us yearning for even the briefest hint of spring. Local gardening aficionados know that's the time to enjoy the height of the camellia season at the Lyman Estate Greenhouses in Waltham.

Thought to be among the oldest surviving greenhouses in the country, the structures on the Lyman Estate are a bucolic destination for plant lovers throughout the year. In fall, at the circa 1804 Grape House, you can luxuriate in the fragrance of blossoming

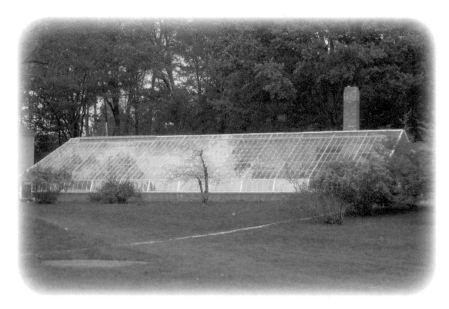

A year-round destination for gardeners

citrus and other exotic fruit trees. In summer, the air there is heavy with the scent of grapes, some of which are descended from George Lyman's collection of rarities, once considered so precious that it's said that only the adults were allowed to eat them.

The 1840 infill greenhouse was originally used to grow roses and cut flowers for the mansion. Now it holds a magnificent collection of orchids, with hundreds of varieties from around the world; you'll almost always find something in bloom there. Yet it's the specimens in the circa 1820 Camellia House that make the Lyman Estate such a desirable winter destination. The plants, some of which are more than a century old, display a profusion of blossoms in just about every shade of red, pink, and white. The paths in the greenhouses are narrow, and weekends can be busy, so I'd advise you to try and get there early.

If you're intrigued by the thought of taking some of that color home, the circa 1930 greenhouse offers plants for sale, and the staff there is very knowledgeable and helpful.

✄ essentials

185 Lyman Street, Waltham, MA 02452

(781) 891-1985

historicnewengland.org/historic-properties/homes/lyman-estate-greenhouses

$ **Greenhouses:** free, though donations suggested. **Guided tours:** Adults: $6; Historic New England members: free

December 15–July 15: Wednesday–Sunday, 9:30 a.m.– 4 p.m. **July 16–December 14:** Wednesday–Saturday, 9:30 a.m.– 4 p.m. Closed most major holidays.
Guided tours: First Wednesday of the month, 11 a.m.–2 p.m. on the hour

n/a

peaceful place 74

MASSACHUSETTS AVENUE BRIDGE MOONRISE

Cambridge, MA (MAP SIX)

CATEGORY ↙ scenic vistas ✪

*J*t's hard to deny that the Mass Ave bridge is one of the busiest thoroughfares in either of the two cities it connects. Four lanes of traffic and two lanes for bicycles—not to mention the pedestrians, in-line skaters, baby strollers, and joggers occupying the sidewalk—can make for a madding crowd. Yet the sweeping river views to the east and west are so breathtaking, especially near sunset, that it's possible to feel peaceful despite the cacophony around you.

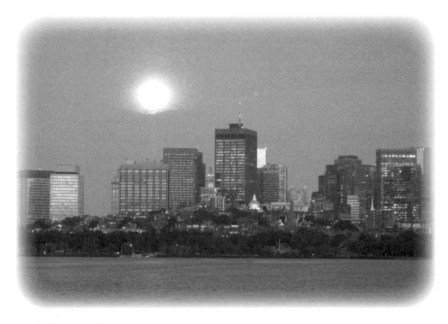

Full moon over Boston

I especially enjoy those early evenings when sailboats and racing sculls still ply the river, the sails turn pink with the setting sun, and Boston begins to sparkle in the twilight. If you time it right, on a clear evening, you can watch the moon rise over the city.

For the best view, head to the Cambridge side of the bridge on the east corner of Memorial Drive. If it's near the time of the month for the full moon, you'll probably run into the regulars who gather with cameras and tripods to capture the first glimpse of that silvery orb as it climbs above the city. They'll be happy to point your gaze in the right direction.

You can stay there, or walk east along the river until you find a quiet place. (There's a bench where you can relax downriver a bit, just across from the MIT Dome.) Feel your mind go free and your spirits soar as the moon rises high enough to send its reflection all the way up the river to meet you. Then walk serenely back across the bridge toward the Back Bay, admiring the moon and cityscape every step of the way.

essentials

📧	Massachusetts Avenue and Memorial Drive, Cambridge, MA 02142
✆	n/a
🌐	n/a
$	Free
🕐	Open 24/7
🚌	T: Bus 1 (Central Square/Cambridge to BU Medical Center) to Beacon Street

peaceful place 75

MASSACHUSETTS COLLEGE OF ART AND DESIGN GALLERIES

Mission Hill, Boston (MAP EIGHT)

CATEGORY ⌣ museums & galleries ✪ ✪ ✪

For many art lovers, the galleries at the Massachusetts College of Art and Design are uncharted territory. But that's part of what makes them such rewarding places for a quiet visit. While there are seven galleries spread throughout the campus, I find three particularly appealing: the Sandra and David Bakalar, the Stephen D. Paine, and the President's Gallery.

As soon as you walk into the building that houses the Bakalar and the Paine, you're greeted by the smell of fresh paint and a palpable energy. This is a place where art is an integral part of life, where it really matters. Established and emerging contemporary artists, as well as students, are the talents behind the exhibitions, which change every month or so. Their work ranges from painting and cutting-edge design to animation and performance art.

The galleries are open and well lighted, with comfortable places to pause while you contemplate the meaning of what you're seeing. Opening receptions can be lively affairs, but at other times, you'll find yourself sharing the space with only a few other visitors. While the atmosphere is stimulating, I usually leave feeling refreshed by the experience.

By contrast, the President's Gallery, located amid the college's executive offices, is a bit more restrained. The reception areas off the 11th-floor main gallery space offer pleasing views of downtown Boston.

If you're seeking a different kind of art experience, spend some time browsing at Mass Art Made, the school's cozy but chic urban boutique. You'll find a juried selection of one-of-a-kind works from jewelry and textiles to ceramics and paintings, all created by Mass Art students, alumni, and faculty. Pieces by established names can be a bit pricey, but those from unknowns or up-and-comers offer the opportunity to support a struggling artist while taking home a treasure.

essentials
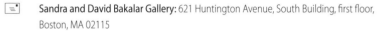

Sandra and David Bakalar Gallery: 621 Huntington Avenue, South Building, first floor, Boston, MA 02115
Stephen D. Paine Gallery: 621 Huntington Avenue, South Building, second floor (enter through Bakalar Gallery), Boston, MA 02115
President's Gallery: 621 Huntington Avenue, Tower Building, 11th floor, Boston, MA 02115
Mass Art Made: 625 Huntington Avenue, Boston, MA 02115

Galleries: (617) 879-7333; **Mass Art Made:** (617) 879-7407

massart.edu
massartmade.com

$ Free, except for purchases

Sandra and David Bakalar and Stephen D. Paine galleries:
Monday–Tuesday and Thursday–Saturday, noon–6 p.m.; Wednesday, noon–8 p.m.
President's Gallery: Monday–Friday, 9 a.m.–5 p.m.
Mass Art Made: Monday–Saturday, 10 a.m.–7 p.m.; Sunday, noon–6 p.m.

T: Green Line, E train, to Longwood Medical

peaceful place 76

MASSACHUSETTS INSTITUTE OF TECHNOLOGY CHAPEL

Cambridge, MA (MAP SIX)

CATEGORY ⌣ spiritual enclaves ✪ ✪ ✪

*H*alf a block off busy Massachusetts Avenue, just beyond the Charles River, is a place I consider to be one of the most sublime spaces in all of greater Boston: Eero Saarinen's Chapel at the Massachusetts Institute of Technology (MIT).

The Saarinen-designed Kresge Auditorium had originally been intended to serve as the campus's religious center. When some of the powers that be at MIT became concerned that the building was too large for that purpose, the architect selected a small corner of what is now called the Kresge Oval as the site for a more intimate structure.

As you walk the path through the birches on the Amherst Street side, you feel as though you're entering a sacred grove, yet nothing prepares you for the serene beauty inside that

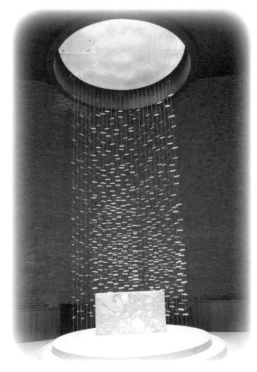

photographed by Christina English

The sculpture screen made of shimmering gold rectangles

cylindrical space. The chapel's simple brick walls were laid in an undulating pattern. (In warmer months, when the moat outside is filled, the small, rounded windows near the floor reflect the play of light and wind on the water outside onto the bricks inside; the effect is almost magical.) The chapel's other main source of illumination is the skylight above the altar. As if to accentuate this, the striking spatial-sculpture-screen of shimmering gold rectangles, designed by Italian artist Harry Bertoia, appears to pour from the space above onto the altar.

One of my favorite times to visit the chapel is during the Wednesday noontime organ concerts held during October, November, February, and March. The Holt-kamp organ, which was designed specifically for this space, provides an almost sculptural presence in the rear of the chapel. So should you position your Saarinen chair to observe the organist or just quietly absorb the way the chapel seems to reverberate with the music? You're welcome to do either—and I usually do both, changing my position between pieces.

essentials

✉   48 Massachusetts Avenue, Building W15, Cambridge, MA 02139

☎   (617) 253-7707

🌐   studentlife.mit.edu/rl

$ Free

🕐   **Chapel:** Daily, 7 a.m.–11 p.m. unless private events are scheduled (check website)
Organ concerts: Check website for seasonal schedule.

🚌   **T:** Bus 1 (Central Square/Cambridge to BU Medical Center) to MIT

peaceful place 77

McCORMICK GALLERY, BOSTON ARCHITECTURAL COLLEGE

Back Bay, Boston (MAP ONE)

CATEGORY ∴ museums & galleries ✪ ✪

*I*n most galleries, the work you see represents an artist's completed vision. The exhibits on display at the Boston Architectural College's McCormick Gallery are often about possibility: how should one best preserve a historic site? How are new technologies informing architectural design? How does one create landscapes for both aesthetics and sustainability? To some, questions of this nature may not seem inherently peaceful. However, I usually leave the McCormick Gallery feeling refreshed by the opportunity to explore new ways of thinking and seeing.

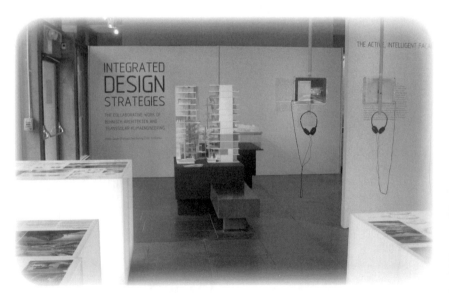

Exhibits on sustainability and historic preservation

The gallery occupies a small space on the ground floor of the college's main building on Newbury Street. There's usually something interesting to see, and the public is always welcome. (For a listing of exhibits, look under "Experience the BAC" on the school's website, cited in "essentials," below.)

Unless a special event is scheduled, the exhibit area never seems to get too crowded, and comfortable benches allow gallerygoers to sit and reflect on the ideas presented here. At times, the exhibits are interactive, and you're welcome to post your responses to the questions that are being posed.

With its big windows facing both Hereford and Newbury streets, McCormick Gallery can be a relaxing spot to pause and do some quiet people-watching after a busy day of working, shopping, or gallery hopping.

↵ essentials

📧 320 Newbury Street, Boston, MA 02115

📞 (617) 262-5000

🌐 the-bac.edu

💲 Free

🕐 Open only when school is in session. Monday–Thursday, 8 a.m.–10:30 p.m.; Friday, 8 a.m.–9 p.m.; Saturday, 9 a.m.–5 p.m.; Sunday, noon–7 p.m.

🚊 T: Green Line, B, C, or D train, to Hynes Auditorium

peaceful place 78

MILLENNIUM PARK

West Roxbury, Boston (MAP EIGHT)

CATEGORY ↙ outdoor habitats ⭐

*M*illennium Park is a reverse of that old magician's "now you see it, now you don't" trick. In its previous life as the West Roxbury landfill, it was a no-man's-land. Now it's among the city's most popular and most-visited parks. And why not? It offers panoramic views from the Blue Hills all the way to downtown Boston. There are also myriad athletic fields, play spaces for kids, and lots of places for picnicking, kite flying, and dog walking.

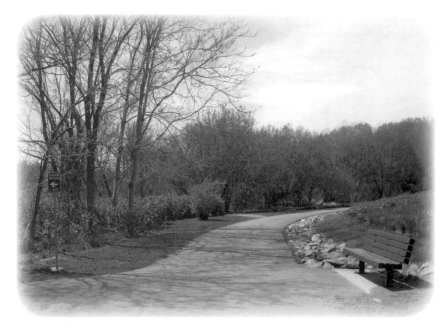

Down the riverside nature trail, especially appealing for birding

Of course, there are enticements for those of us who usually avoid this kind of open-space park. At its eastern edge is an area referred to as the Dump Shoreline Urban Wild, a rather ungracious way of saying that the Charles River winds along here on its way to Boston. There, you'll find a nature trail that echoes with birdsong while offering opportunities to commune with herons and other marsh-loving wildlife.

Feel the call of the river? There's a boat ramp here where you can put in a canoe or kayak and paddle on this gentle stretch of the Charles—or go all the way downstream to the canoe landing at Nahanton Park in Newton. (The Charles River Watershed Association has published a guide to the river from Bellingham to Boston. See **charlesriver.org.**)

If the nature walk tempts you to meander farther, look for the bridge over the Sawmill Brook that leads to the Brook Farm Historic Site, home of the Transcendentalist community that counted Nathaniel Hawthorne, Ralph Waldo Emerson, and Margaret Fuller among its members and frequent visitors. Here you'll find a more pastoral experience than at Millennium, as you wander through woodlands, wetlands, and gently rolling fields. (The Gardens at Gethsemane Cemetery site also occupies a portion of this property. The staff there welcomes visitors.)

The properties described here (and on pages 117 and 121) are often referred to as part of the city of Newton's system of parks and conservation lands. To learn more, visit the website of the Newton Conservators (see "essentials," below).

⌖ essentials

⌗ Off Veterans of Foreign Wars Parkway at Gardner Street, West Roxbury, MA 02132

☏ (617) 635-4505   ⌖ newtonconservators.org/34millennium.htm

$ Free   ☉ Daily, sunrise–sunset

⛝ T: Orange Line to Forest Hills, then Bus 36 to Gardner Street (Buses run infrequently; check with driver.)

peaceful place 79

MONASTERY OF THE SOCIETY OF SAINT JOHN THE EVANGELIST

Cambridge, MA (MAP SIX)

CATEGORY ⌣ spiritual enclaves ✪ ✪ ✪

*W*ho doesn't sometimes yearn for a little silence, serenity, or spirituality in the midst of an over-scheduled life? Just steps from the bustle and clamor of Harvard

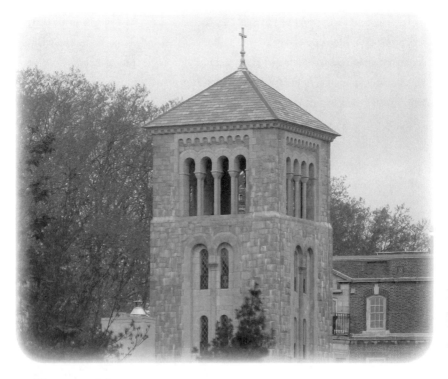

The monastery bell tower

Square, you will find a monastery where the brothers live in a world of prayer and contemplation. Best of all, you're invited to experience that tranquility yourself for a few minutes, an hour, or even a couple of days.

For 75 years, the Monastery of the Society of Saint John the Evangelist has stood in this location, near the banks of the Charles River. The circa 1936 French Romanesque chapel, with its limestone pillars and marble floors, is said to be one of architect Ralph Adams Cram's masterpieces. Here, where the brothers chant prayers several times a day, you're welcome to enjoy some peaceful reflection 6 a.m.–9 p.m., whether you choose to attend a service, spend some time in silent meditation, or just sit and admire the light from the beautiful stained glass rose window.

Looking to really get away from it all for a night or two or more? The monastery's comfortable guesthouse, with its 12 single bedrooms, library, and soothing garden, offers visitors a calming space for a personal retreat. You're free to structure your time to meet your needs, joining the brothers in their daily round of worship, silence, and meals as much or as little as you please.

⌣ essentials

☰ 34 Concord Avenue, Cambridge, MA 02138
Chapel: 980 Memorial Drive, Cambridge, MA 02138

☎ (617) 876-3037

🌐 ssje.org

$ **Service attendance:** free, though donations suggested. **Guesthouse single room, with meals:** $100 per night

🕐 **Chapel:** Tuesday–Saturday, 6 a.m.–9 p.m.; Sunday, 6:30 a.m.–5 p.m.
For service schedule: See website above.

🚃 **T:** Red Line to Harvard

peaceful place 80

MOTHERS' WALK, ROSE F. KENNEDY GREENWAY
Waterfront District, Boston (MAP THREE)

CATEGORY ↙ urban surprises ✪

*I*n 2008, the last of Boston's hulking Central Artery was demolished, courtesy of the somewhat controversial Big Dig tunnel project. In its place, the winding, mile-long Rose F. Kennedy Greenway came into being. While naysayers seem to focus only on the projects that have so far failed to come to fruition—the winter garden, a museum, and a new YMCA—I prefer to celebrate what has been realized. In addition to the Boston Harbor Islands visitor center, a carousel, and a couple of dramatic fountains, one of the most interesting spots is the gently meandering Mothers' Walk. This peaceful

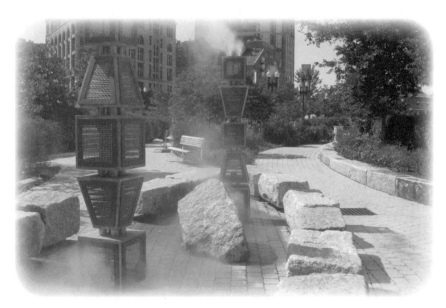

Ross Miller's motion-activated sculpture Harbor Fog

destination is located between High and State streets on the Atlantic Avenue and Wharf District side of the greenway.

On a nice day, a stroll here can be a pleasant pastime. I enjoy noting the names and messages inscribed on the pavers that line the walkway. I like to contemplate the diversity of not just the mothers but also fathers, daughters, sons, mentors, and others—both living and not—who are honored here. (My own mother's paver, which reads "With love to Mary Jane Schweikart," is about 20 feet in, near the residences at the Boston Harbor Hotel.)

At the corner of Atlantic Avenue and State Street, you can view the pavers saluting members of the Kennedy family, including Caroline, Jacqueline, Maria Shriver, and Rose herself.

essentials

- Atlantic Avenue between High and State streets, Boston, MA 02109

- (617) 262-5000

- rosekennedygreenway.org (Click "Visit" on the drop-down menus, then "Greenway Parks," then "Wharf District" for the specific "Mothers' Walk" section.)

- $ Free

- Open 24/7

- T: Red Line to South Station; Blue Line to Aquarium

peaceful place 81

MOUNT AUBURN CEMETERY

Cambridge, MA (MAP SIX)

CATEGORY ⌄ enchanting walks ✪ ✪ ✪

*O*n early mornings in spring, especially on weekends, birders imitate the feathered creatures and flock to Mount Auburn Cemetery. Heaven help you if you come between them and, say, a Cape May warbler. (On the other hand, should you want to find that bird, you'll have dozens of people eager to help you.) No matter. With 175 acres and more than 10 miles of roads and paths, the grounds are large and varied enough to offer tranquility and sensory delight in every season.

Founded in 1831, Mount Auburn quickly became the model for the kind of land-scaped sanctuary that served as an arboretum as well as a final resting place. It has its share

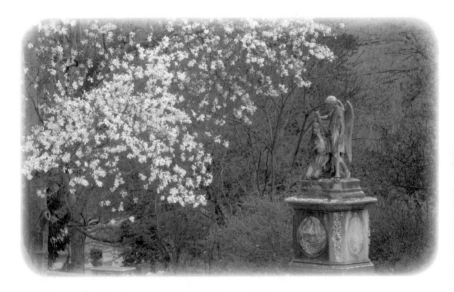

Mount Auburn in spring, when it is particularly breathtaking

of famous "residents," including poet Henry Wadsworth Longfellow, cookbook author Fannie Farmer, writer Bernard Malamud, and engineer Buckminster Fuller (inventor of the geodesic dome). While the cemetery offers tours of its statuary, plantings, and the graves of the famous, I find it more peaceful to amble about on my own. (That way you're more likely to encounter one of Mount Auburn's living inhabitants: a fox, owl, or even the red-tailed hawk that seems to delight in swooping down on unwary visitors.)

The natural beauty of Mount Auburn, with its hills, dells, knolls, and ponds, inspires contemplative wandering. There are nearly 6,000 trees—600 varieties of 75 genera, most labeled and recorded—as well as some 250 species of shrubs and ground covers. A walk along Indian Ridge in spring is an olfactory delight as scents of magnolia, viburnum, lilac, and crab apple blossoms mingle in the air.

The wonderfully secluded Consecration Dell is one of my favorite places to linger momentarily, especially if I happen to catch the haunting sound of a wood thrush singing. (The pond there is also home to one of the largest breeding colonies of spotted salamanders in eastern Massachusetts.) Equally serene, as long as there's not too much traffic on nearby Mount Auburn Street, is Spruce Knoll, the new contemplation garden created amid a glade of towering spruce trees by the well-known landscape designer Julie Moir Messervy. Also plan to visit the Mount Auburn's Cemetery Washington Tower, another peaceful spot (see page 178).

⌣ essentials
_____

⌨   580 Mount Auburn Street, Cambridge, MA 02138   ✆   (617) 547-7105

🌐   mountauburn.org $ Free

🕐   **October–April:** Daily, 8 a.m.–5 p.m. **May–September:** Daily, 8 a.m.–7 p.m.

🚌   **T:** Bus 71 (Harvard to Watertown Square) to Homer Avenue

peaceful place 82

MOUNT AUBURN CEMETERY, WASHINGTON TOWER

Cambridge, MA (MAP SIX)

CATEGORY ⌣ scenic vistas ⭐

*A*t 125 feet above sea level, Washington Tower provides an incomparable panorama of the Charles River, Cambridge, downtown Boston, and beyond. And that's before you climb the 90-some granite steps to the top of the 62-foot tower. As someone who suffers a bit from vertigo, I have to admit that the 150-year-old staircase

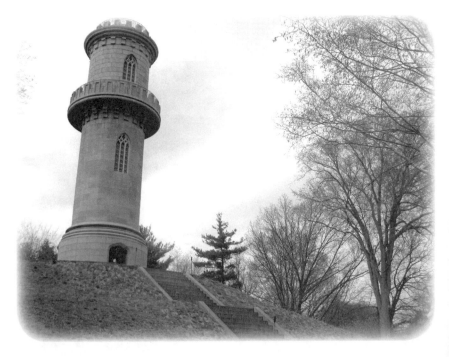

The granite tower, built in 1852–54

is not quite my cup of tea. But the anticipation of the view always beckons me onward anyway, and I've never been disappointed once I've reached my goal.

Unless it's crowded at the top—a good reason to avoid midday on weekends—plan to spend some time to savor not just the city toward the horizon but also the incredible natural landscape that spreads out beneath you. You're getting a bit of the bird's-eye view that has made Mount Auburn one of the East Coast's most famous and reliable spots from which to experience the spring avian migration.

Once you're safely back on terra firma, stop to admire the butterfly garden planted around the tower's base. I make sure to visit this spot whenever I'm taking a walk around Mount Auburn Cemetery, which is a peaceful destination in itself (see page 176). Because it's possible to drive up Mountain Avenue to the base of the tower, it's worth a special trip near the end of the day during fall and winter. In those seasons and at that time, the leaves or snow pick up the sunset colors, and Cambridge and Boston sparkle like jewels in the treetops below.

essentials

☞ 580 Mount Auburn Street, Cambridge, MA 02138

☏ (617) 547-7105

🌐 mountauburn.org

$ Free

🕐 **October–April:** Daily, 8 a.m.–5 p.m. **May–September:** Daily, 8 a.m.–7 p.m.

🚌 **T:** Bus 71 (Harvard to Watertown Square) to Homer Avenue

peaceful place 83

MOUNT AUBURN STREET, MIDDLE EASTERN MARKETS
Watertown, MA (MAP SIX)
CATEGORY ⌣ shops & services ⭐

or foodies with a hankering for Middle Eastern flavors, the half block or so between 569 and 599 Mount Auburn Street is like finding the Holy Grail. Just walk through the door at Massis Bakery and Specialty Foodstore, Sevan Bakery, or Arax Market; close your eyes; and inhale the captivating aromas. Olives. Spices. Citrus. Sweets. Listen to the music and snatches of conversation in Armenian or Lebanese. Most of all, contemplate the exotic tastes that you're about to savor.

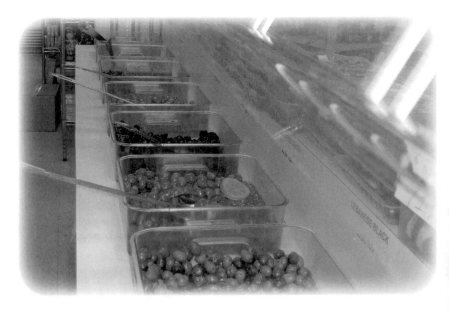

A food lover's delight

I usually wander through all three stores before I decide what tempting treats to sample, and it's never an easy decision. Sevan and Massis, both Armenian bakeries, have large cases full of homemade sweet and savory pastries. Arax, the Lebanese grocery store, has fresh-made pita delivered every day. Sevan has 17 kinds of cured olives, and Massis and Arax almost as many. In all three stores, there are pickles of every description and more spice mixtures and candies than you could ever imagine.

In addition to cheeses from Egypt, Syria, and Bulgaria, you'll also find dried fruits and the freshest nuts in town, plus an enticing variety of coffees and teas. For the more adventurous shopper who desires an exotic pipe, Arax stocks an intriguing selection of hookahs. Take home some of Massis's amazingly spicy homemade hummus and other mezes for a cold supper or picnic. You'll feel as though you've just spent a pleasant day in Istanbul, Beirut, or Yerevan, despite world tensions.

∿ essentials

📧 **Massis Bakery:** 569 Mount Auburn Street, Watertown, MA 02472
    Sevan Bakery: 599 Mount Auburn Street, Watertown, MA 02472
    Arax Market: 585 Mount Auburn Street, Watertown, MA 02472

📞 **Massis Bakery:** (617) 924-0537
    Sevan Bakery: (617) 924-3243
    Arax Market: (617) 924-3399

🌐 massisbakery.com
    sevanboston.com

$ Free, except for purchases

🕐 **Massis and Sevan bakeries:** Monday–Saturday, 8 a.m.–8 p.m.
    Arax Market: Monday–Saturday, 9 a.m.–8 p.m.; Sunday, 11 a.m.–4 p.m.

🚌 **T:** Bus 71 (Harvard to Watertown Square) to Adams Street

peaceful place 84

MUSEUM OF FINE ARTS, BOSTON

The Fenway, Boston (MAP FIVE)

CATEGORY ⌣ museums & galleries ✪

*E*ach year, the Museum of Fine Arts (MFA), Boston welcomes more than a million
visitors through its grand entrances off Huntington Avenue and The Fenway.
This can present a challenge to anyone looking forward to an intimate encounter with
the museum's remarkable collection, particularly the always popular Claude Monets,
Pierre-Auguste Renoirs, and other Impressionist paintings. (The recent opening of the
new Art of the Americas wing means that those who wish to spend some quiet time viewing such beloved works as John Singer Sargent's *The Daughters of Edward Darley Boit* and
Childe Hassam's *Boston Common at Twilight* will be similarly tested.)

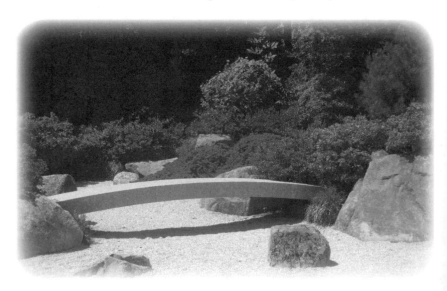

A restful place at Tenshin-En

Not to worry. The MFA offers myriad places where you can go to escape the crowds and refresh your spirit. One of my favorites is the Japanese Buddhist Temple Room, a softly lit space designed in 1909 to evoke the temple of Hōryūji, one of the oldest in Japan. Sink onto a bench and take a few minutes to commune silently with Amida, the Buddha of Infinite Light; and Dainichi, the Buddha of Infinite Illumination.

If a calming outdoor oasis is more to your liking, search out Tenshin-En, the museum's 10,000-square-foot Japanese rock garden. The entrance, marked by a magnificent wooden gate, is outside on the Museum Road side of the building, near the corner of The Fenway. (Be prepared to show your proof of admission payment.)

Wednesday–Friday, the MFA is open until 9:45 p.m. Even on Wednesdays, when the admission fee is voluntary after 4 p.m., I find that the crowds begin to thin out after 7:30 or so, when most people start contemplating dinner. That's also a quiet time to visit the bookshop, which offers one of the city's best selections of art, architecture, and design titles.

Those who find sketching to be a relaxing activity will enjoy Drawing in the Galleries on Wednesday evenings. Sketch live models or objects from the museum's collection while picking up a few insights into drawing techniques.

↝ essentials

465 Huntington Avenue, Boston, MA 02115

(617) 267-9300   mfa.org

$ Adults: $22; seniors age 65 and older and students age 18 and older: $20; **children ages 7–17:** $10, but free Monday–Friday after 3 p.m., Saturday–Sunday, and Boston public school holidays; **children age 6 and younger and members:** free; **Wednesday after 4 p.m.:** free, though suggested donation of $22.

Monday–Tuesday and Saturday–Sunday, 10 a.m.–4:45 p.m.; Wednesday–Friday, 10 a.m.–9:45 p.m. **Drawing in the Galleries:** Most Wednesdays, 6–9 p.m. Check the website under "Programs" and then "Gallery Activities/Tours" for details.

T: Green Line, E train, to Museum of Fine Arts

peaceful place 85

NEW ENGLAND AQUARIUM, HARBOR SEALS

Waterfront District, Boston (MAP THREE)

CATEGORY ↶ urban surprises ⭐

'll never forget my first exploration around the four-story giant ocean tank at the New England Aquarium. It was during my early days in working as a "creative" in Boston advertising, and some TV or radio station had taken over the whole building for a party. Most people hung out around the bars and food tables downstairs, so some friends and I were able to escape the crowd and wander around the upper levels to our heart's content, admiring the sharks, rays, and other sea creatures living there.

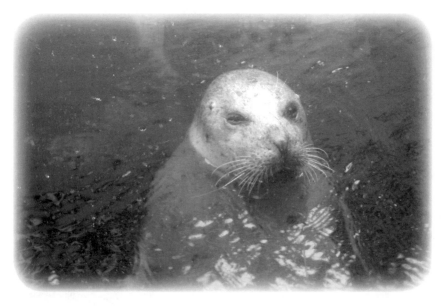

A harbor seal ready for a nap

The challenge at the aquarium is not finding something to delight you; it's finding a time when you won't feel overwhelmed by the cacophony of other visitors. For that reason, it's best to avoid weekends and mornings, if possible. Weekday midafternoons frequently offer sublime moments of calm, as you watch the sea turtles float by in their seemingly meditative state.

One of my secret pleasures is the harbor seal exhibit outside on the aquarium's Front Plaza. When I worked in the Financial District, I'd frequently go there for a late lunch hour and spend a few moments communing with Amelia, Smoke, Reggae, and the others as they swam, sunned, and played. I always walked back to the office feeling surprisingly refreshed and restored.

⌣ essentials

📧 1 Central Wharf, Boston, MA 02110

📞 (617) 973-5200

🌐 neaq.org

$ **Adults:** $22.95; **children ages 3–11:** $15.95; **seniors age 60 and older:** $20.95; **children age 2 and younger and members:** free. **Harbor seal exhibit:** free. Tickets for the Aquarium's IMAX theater and Whale Watches are available separately and in combination with the aquarium admission.

🕐 **July–Labor Day:** Sunday–Thursday, 9 a.m.-6 p.m.; Friday–Saturday, 9 a.m.–7 p.m.; **July 4,** 9 a.m.–7 p.m.; **Labor Day,** 9 a.m.–6 p.m.
Day after Labor Day–June: Monday–Friday, 9 a.m.-5 p.m.; Saturday–Sunday and most holidays, 9 a.m.–6 p.m. Closed Thanksgiving and December 25; opens at noon on January 1.

🚉 **T:** Blue Line to Aquarium

peaceful place 86

NEW ENGLAND WILDFLOWER SOCIETY, GARDEN IN THE WOODS

Framingham, MA (MAP NINE)

CATEGORY ⌣ outdoor habitats ✪ ✪

*J*n May, wetlands, woodlands, hillsides, and mountains throughout New England erupt with blooms, both subtle and showy. Unfortunately, busy lives too often leave little time to search out and appreciate this fleeting beauty. That's when a trip to the Garden in the Woods is in order.

The 45-acre garden, begun in 1931 by landscape architect Will Curtis, re-creates a wide range of habitats where rare and endangered plants native to New England can flourish. Now under the auspices of the New England Wildflower Society, the nation's

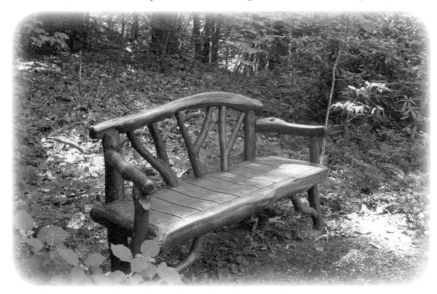

A spot for quiet contemplation

oldest plant-conservation organization, Garden in the Woods is home to more than 1,000 native plant species.

To truly appreciate the diversity of plant life here, I recommend one of the guided walks, especially during peak blooming times. However, peacefulness can be found here in every season, and if that's what you're seeking, I suggest you amble off on your own among the four nature trails.

I'm particularly fond of Hop Brook Trail, which meanders along and over a gurgling brook. Here and there, you'll find a convenient log on which to linger and be lulled by the calming sounds of brook and birdsong, while neon emerald- and sapphire-colored dragonflies dart about. At the top of Beech Grove, where Hop Brook Trail meets the main trail, there's a restful wooden bench for you to pause and admire the view or do some woodland sketches.

To extend your range, head for the Ridge and Lady's-slipper trails, which wind through the pine and oak woodlands at the northwestern edge of the property. If you are there in August, be sure to stroll through the meadow area between the Lady's-slipper and Hop Brook trails; it's a haven for butterflies, and the plants that attract them are at their peak blooming time that month.

↙ essentials

⌨ 180 Hemenway Road, Framingham, MA 01701   (508) 877-7630

🌐 newfs.org (Type "Garden in the Woods" into the search box.)

$ Adults: $10; seniors age 65 and older: $7; children ages 3–17: $5; children age 2 and younger and members: free

🕐 April 15–October: Tuesday–Sunday and holiday Mondays, 9 a.m.–5 p.m.; last admission at 4:30 p.m. (April 15–July 4: Thursday, 8 a.m.–8 p.m.; last admission at 7:30 p.m.) Guided walk: Tuesday–Friday, 10 a.m.; Saturday–Sunday, 2 p.m.

🚘 n/a

peaceful place 87

NORMAN B. LEVENTHAL PARK

Post Office Square, Financial District, Boston (MAP THREE)

CATEGORY ↙ parks & gardens ✪ ✪

" hey paved paradise, and put up a parking lot," or so sang Joni Mitchell in her hit 1970s ballad. Happily, that's the opposite of what happened at Post Office Square in Boston's Financial District. Here, a decrepit concrete parking structure was torn down and replaced by an underground garage (dubbed the "Garage Mahal" because of its prices and amenities), and the street-level space was transformed into the bucolic Norman B. Leventhal Park. This 1.7-acre space contains more than 125 trees, shrubs, and plants. (The largest trees, a hybrid red oak, an eastern arborvitae, and two giant western arborvitae, are on permanent loan from the Arnold Arboretum, another peaceful place, which appears on page 8.)

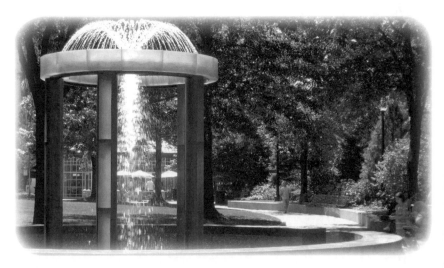

The fountain at Post Office Square

The park's 0.5-acre lawn is so lush that the groundskeeper at Fenway Park must be green with envy. Not only are you welcome to sit on the grass, but if you do, one of the helpful park attendants is also likely to hand you a cushion so you don't stain your clothes. Someone was even thoughtful enough to install Wi-Fi!

I haven't experienced such a rendezvous myself, but the scuttlebutt is that the park is a great place for single 24- to 32-year-old professionals to meet. Apparently more than flowers blossom here in Post Office Square.

Most days, I prefer the north end of the park. It's far enough from the bustle created by the patrons of Sip Café, yet near enough to hear the live music at lunchtime in the summer. Or sit close to *Immanent Circumstance*, the commanding glass-and-bronze sculpture fountain by Howard Ben Tré, and close your eyes as the sound of cascading water completely obscures the noise of the traffic.

On nice weekends, when other Boston destinations can get a little busy, Post Office Square is a superb spot to escape the crowds. For birding enthusiasts, spring and fall are excellent times to visit, as the park is a frequent resting place for passing warblers, thrushes, and other songbirds.

✌ essentials

🖃 Bounded by Franklin, Pearl, Milk, and Congress streets, Boston, MA 02110

📞 **Friends of Post Office Square:** (617) 423-1500; **Sip Café:** (617) 338-3080

🌍 normanbleventhalpark.org; sipboston.com   **$** Free

🕐 Daily, 6 a.m.–9 p.m. **Sip Café:** December–March: Monday–Friday, 6:30 a.m.–5 p.m. April–November: Monday–Friday, 6:30 a.m.–6 p.m.

🚈 **T:** Orange Line to State or Downtown Crossing; Red Line to Downtown Crossing; Silver Line or Commuter Rail to South Station

peaceful place 88

NORTH END SHOPPING

North End, Boston (MAP THREE)

CATEGORY ⌣ shops & services ✪

*W*hen locals think about peaceful spots in Boston, the North End is probably not the first place that comes to mind. Here, you're more likely to encounter tourists and traffic than to find tranquility. Yet, that doesn't mean that you have to sacrifice serenity to enjoy this neighborhood's genuine Italian charm.

I recommend that you head away from Hanover Street and stroll along Salem Street, away from the Rose F. Kennedy Greenway. As you walk past the cafés and shops here, you're likely to hear snatches of conversation that make you feel as though you've wandered into a small town in southern Italy. Farther up Salem, you'll come to Bova's Bakery. (You may catch the scent of warm bread before you even see the shop.) The bakery, now run by the third generation of Bovas, has been in this same location since 1932. It's open 24 hours a day, so if you're looking for a fresh-baked *pane rotondo* for breakfast, a picnic, or a midnight snack, this is the place to come. Bova's also makes a superb cannoli— which is probably why you never see locals waiting in those long lines at Mike's.

Among the pleasures of the North End is the possibility of finding authentic Italian specialty foods. One of my favorite purveyors is Salumeria Italiana. I think its friendly little shop on Richmond Street has the neighborhood's best selection of salami, cheeses, olives, and artisanal pasta, not to mention olive oils and vinegars. I love to while away some time there, imagining all the wonderful things that I can put on an antipasto platter—and I rarely leave empty handed.

DePasquale's is a relative newcomer to the neighborhood, but its homemade pasta— made fresh on the premises—is available in more than 50 shapes and sizes. Not sure what variety to serve with which sauce? Just ask the pasta specialist.

After shopping in the North End, it's traditional to unwind at a café with an espresso, grappa, or *limonata*. (Or red or white wine, if you prefer.) Skip the places where soccer fans gather on game days and head to Caffé Vittoria, said to be the city's oldest Italian café. (It opened in 1929.) The hand-painted murals and family photos on the wall give it a comfortable, old-world ambience. The most tranquil tables are in the rear.

⌣ essentials

▣ **Bova's Bakery:** 134 Salem Street, Boston, MA 02113
   Salumeria Italiana: 151 Richmond Street, Boston, MA 02109
   DePasquale's Homemade Pasta Shoppe: 66A Cross Street, Boston, MA 02113
   Caffé Vittoria: 290–296 Hanover Street, Boston, MA 02113

☎ **Bova's Bakery:** (617) 523-5601
   Salumeria Italiana: (617) 523-8743
   DePasquale's Homemade Pasta Shoppe: (617) 248-9629
   Caffé Vittoria: (617) 227-7606

🌐 bovabakeryboston.com
   salumeriaitaliana.com
   homemade-pasta.com
   vittoriacaffe.com

$ Free, except for purchases

🕐 **Bova's Bakery:** Open 24/7
   Salumeria Italiana: Monday–Saturday, 8 a.m.–7 p.m.; Sunday, 10 a.m.–4 p.m.
   DePasquale's Homemade Pasta Shoppe: Monday–Thursday, 10 a.m.–8 p.m.; Friday, 10 a.m.–10 p.m.; Saturday, 9 a.m.–10 p.m.; Sunday, 10 a.m.–8 p.m.
   Caffé Vittoria: Sunday–Thursday, 7 a.m.–midnight; Friday–Saturday, 7 a.m.–12:30 a.m.

🚌 **T:** Green Line or Orange Line to Haymarket

peaceful place 89

NORTH POINT PARK

Charles River Reservation, East Cambridge, MA (MAP SEVEN)

CATEGORY ⌣ parks & gardens ⭐

*T*here's something appropriate about the wild, meadowlike feel of this park. It sits on what was once called the "lost half mile," that area on the east side of the Charles River locks, where the river seemed to disappear and the cities on either side faded away into a maze of rail yards, highways, and industrial wastelands.

Talk about urban renewal! Now there are winding paths, where masses of bulbs, grasses, roses, and other perennials line the banks of little waterways that lead out to the rediscovered river. Secluded spots entice you to groves of birch and linden trees, benches

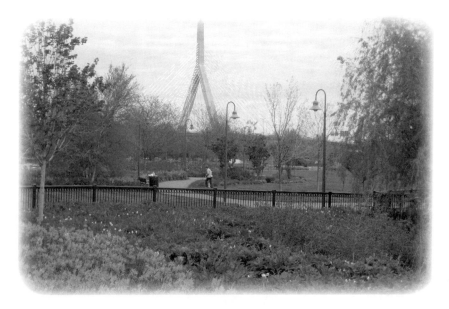

The view toward the Leonard P. Zakim Bridge

galore, and lush grassy areas for picnicking, lounging in the sun, or just laying back and watching boats and trains go by. For the kids, there's not one but two play areas. For adults, there's a handy ramp for launching a kayak or canoe and heading off for a lazy paddle. And the sunsets from both water and land are spectacular. The only catch? Parking is not very convenient.

In some respects, this is also the *last* half mile—the pilings are in place and work is in progress for the pedestrian and bicycle bridge that will connect North Point to Paul Revere and City Square parks in Charlestown and the HarborWalk beyond. (A skate park is also planned for that area, raising some concerns as to how the serenity of North Point will be affected.)

Nonetheless, once the bridge is completed, one will be able to bike or walk the entire length of the Charles River Reservation—from Watertown through the city and out onto the HarborWalk—as far as it stretches in each direction.[*] Imagine the possibilities for finding your pockets of tranquility then!

[*]*Note:* Don't have a bike? Check out New Balance Hubway, Boston's terrific new bike-sharing system. Learn more at **thehubway.com.**

✌ essentials

⌐▪⌐   Off Monsignor O'Brien Highway at Museum Way, Boston, MA 02141

📞   n/a

🌐   mass.gov/dcr/parks/charlesRiver (Click on "Plan Your Visit," and scroll to "North Point Park.")

$ Free

🕐   Daily, sunrise–sunset

🚌   T: Green Line, any train, to Science Park or Lechmere

peaceful place 90

OCEANIC HOUSE, STAR ISLAND

Isles of Shoals, NH (MAP TEN)

CATEGORY ↙ day trips & overnights ✪ ✪

*C*an't resist the siren song of the sea? Ten miles off the New Hampshire coast, among the rugged Isles of Shoals, you'll find a haven for indulging that passion: the Oceanic House at Star Island. The boat ride on *Uncle Oscar* from Rye Harbor to Gosport Harbor (short for God's port) takes only 45 minutes, but you'll feel as though you've been transported to an earlier era.

More than 100 years old, the Oceanic harkens back to those days when New Englanders in need of rest, relaxation, and relief from summer heat flocked to the grand hotels that dotted the coastline. Today, the Oceanic has a rustic, almost camplike feel, with rocking chairs on the big wraparound porch, a dining room where everyone eats family style,

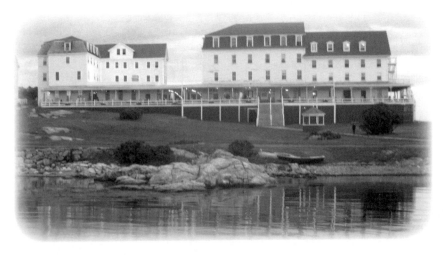

Picture-perfect from the era of grand hotels

and relatively spartan guest rooms. Bathrooms are communal, and showers are available only at set times, every other day. Don't bother to bring your laptop; not only is there no Wi-Fi, but most rooms also lack even electrical outlets. (There *is* cell phone service, though use is discouraged on the porch and in the first-floor common areas. And if you must go online, you can use one of the computers near the gift shop, for a fee.)

What you give up in luxury is more than made up for by the restorative powers of the island. Sunrises, sunsets, and moonrises seem profoundly moving, as is the star-filled sky. At night, you'll be lulled to sleep by the sound of the ocean and the foghorn at White Island Light. By day, take rejuvenating walks or refreshing swims, or relax and read on the porch.

Whether you come for one of the conferences or workshops given under the auspices of the Star Island Corporation, or for a personal retreat, you can socialize with fellow islanders as much or as little as you desire. Regardless of your spiritual proclivities, one thing you'll want to do at least once is participate in the nightly, lantern-lit silent processions to the circa 1800 stone chapel.

There's a chant that Shoalers, as Star Island devotees are called, recite to those leaving the island: "S-T-A-R, S-T-A-R, Oceanic, Oceanic, you'll come back." The reply: "S-T-A-R, S-T-A-R, Oceanic, Oceanic, we will come back." And I predict that you will.

essentials

✉ c/o Star Island Corporation, Morton-Benedict House, 30 Middle Street, Portsmouth, NH 03801

☎ (603) 430-6272; **island phone:** (603) 601-0832   🌐 starisland.org

$ **Conferences price:** $75–$225, one-time fee per person, plus $130–$203 per person, per night, for room and board. **Personal retreats:** $70–$132 per person, per night, for room and board

🕐 **Oceanic House:** Mid-June–mid-September
Grounds (for day guests): Mid-June–Labor Day, 8 a.m.–sunset

🚌 Boat transportation to and from the island can be arranged at ryeharborcruises.com or islesofshoals.com.

peaceful place 91

OLD SOUTH CHURCH, CHORUS PRO MUSICA SING

Back Bay, Boston (MAP ONE)

CATEGORY ᴗ urban surprises ✪ ✪

onday evenings in August, you'll find an eclectic crowd entering the Old South Church on the corner of Boylston and Dartmouth streets in the Back Bay. You may want to be among them. If you are, a hint of excitement fills the air as you walk up to the fourth-floor Guild Room. You're about to participate in a grand Boston tradition: the Chorus pro Musica Summer Sings.

Under the expert guidance of Chorus pro Musica's musical director, you'll rehearse a major choral work by composers such as Bach, Mozart, Brahms, or Verdi for the first hour and a half. After a short break, you'll reconvene and perform the work in full. There's no audience, no stage, and only a piano accompaniment—though professionals sing the solo parts.

Even if you can't really carry a tune, there's something powerful about sitting in the midst of all those voices, feeling the music of some of the greatest sacred works of all time reverberating inside of and around you. You'll walk back out into the summer night feeling exhilarated and restored. No reservations are required. Refreshments and scores are provided. The hall is air-conditioned and wheelchair accessible. Altogether, it's a perfect recipe for a fulfilling experience that inspires calmness.

⌣ essentials

✉ **Old South Church:** 645 Boylston Street, Boston, MA 02116

☎ **Old South Church:** (617) 536-1970; **Summer Sings:** (617) 267-7442

🌐 Visit oldsouth.org for more about the church.
Visit choruspromusica.org for details about year-round performances.
E-mail chorusinfo@choruspromusica.org to inquire about the Summer
Sings schedule.

$ $8 per person, per event; discounts for seniors and students

🕐 First four Mondays in August, 7:30–10 p.m.

🚍 **T:** Green Line, any train, to Copley

peaceful place 92

154 LOUNGE, BACK BAY HOTEL

Back Bay, Boston (MAP ONE)
CATEGORY ⌣ quiet tables ✪ ✪

*N*ext time you have the occasion to slip out of the office and meet an important client for coffee, you might want to consider the Back Bay Hotel's 154 Lounge. This tranquil spot just off the lobby is one of Boston's best-kept secrets, so it makes a big impression. You can sink into one of the colorful overstuffed couches or easy chairs and sit in front of the gas fireplace, or pick a window seat overlooking the outdoor patio on Berkeley Street.

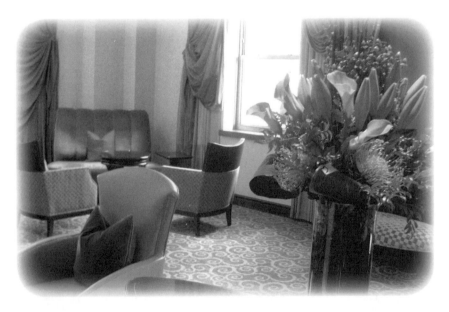

One of Boston's best-kept secrets

While the menu is simple—mostly pastries, yogurt parfaits, and other light morning fare—the setting hints at a bit of modernist sophistication that's missing from the typical Boston breakfast place. As a nod to the fact that the building once housed the city's old police headquarters, the bar on the hotel's ground floor is called Cuffs.

The hotel is happy to share its Wi-Fi network with nonguests visiting the lounge, and there are newspapers provided to keep you occupied until your own guest arrives—or while you relax there by yourself.

In the evenings, the 154 Lounge (named for the address at the hotel's Berkeley Street entrance) becomes an out-of-the-way spot to enjoy cocktails and share a charcuterie or cheese platter. Between times, there's no food or beverage service, but the comfortable space still offers a welcoming retreat, particularly on a chilly day, when the fireplace beckons.

⌣ essentials

⊡   154 Lounge, Back Bay Hotel, 350 Stuart Street, Boston, MA 02116

✆   (617) 266-7200

🌐   doylecollection.com/locations/boston_hotels.aspx

$ **Coffee:** $2.75; **wine and beer:** from $8; **appetizer platters:** $10–$12

🕐   **Breakfast:** Daily, 6–11 a.m. **Cocktails:** Tuesday–Thursday, 5:30–11 p.m.; Friday–Saturday, 5:30 p.m.–1 a.m.

🚋   **T:** Green Line, any train, to Arlington

peaceful place 93

101 MERRIMAC STREET ATRIUM

North Station, Boston (MAP TWO)

CATEGORY ⌣ urban surprises ✪

*O*n dreary Boston winter days, it's fun to plot an escape to someplace sunny and tropical. That's when I try to make a visit to the atrium at 101 Merrimac Street. Walk through the doors and you're greeted by the soothing sound of water from a small fountain. But it's the six-story wall behind that fountain that makes this place so appealing. There, artist Richard Haas has created a soaring, floor-to-ceiling trompe l'oeil mural of a glass-domed winter garden pavilion, overflowing with tropical specimens. The plants in the painting evoke such detail that a botanist could probably identify the genus and species. If you look closely, you'll even spy a solitary parrot flying through the greenery.

As this constitutes the lobby area of a good-size office building, things can get a bit hectic when large numbers of people are entering and exiting the elevator banks. So for the greatest enjoyment of this pleasant illusion, try to drop in midmorning or midafternoon. The tables and chairs provided by the adjoining Au Bon Pain invite sitting with a cup of tea or hot chocolate and absorbing the scenery.

⌣ essentials

▤ 101 Merrimac Street, Boston, MA 02114

🕻 n/a   🌐 n/a $ Free

🕧 Monday–Friday, 6 a.m.–6 p.m.

🚌 T: Orange Line or Green Line, North Station train, to Haymarket or North Station

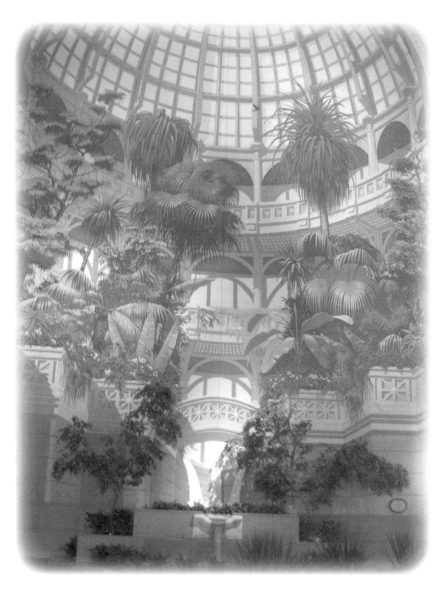

A tropical—painted!—paradise in the heart of downtown Boston

peaceful place 94

PANOPTICON GALLERY

Kenmore Square, Boston (MAP FIVE)

CATEGORY ↙ museums & galleries ⊙ ⊙

*T*he Panopticon Gallery is regarded as one of the oldest fine-art photography galleries in the United States. Since its establishment in 1971, it has moved to a number of places in and around Boston. Almost a decade ago, Panopticon settled into its current space: a smallish, quiet spot just off the main lobby of the Hotel Commonwealth in Kenmore Square.

Because the Panopticon caters to private collectors, museums, and corporations, the photography on display—whether by established artists or by those who are up and

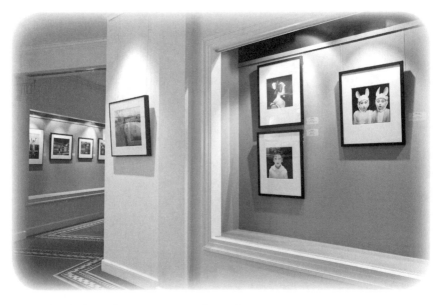

My favorite place in Boston to see top-rate photography

coming—is always of the highest quality. The bench-type seating and light jazz that's usually floating in from the hotel's music system conjure up the perfect atmosphere for contemplating the exhibits, which change about eight times a year. Unless there is an opening reception, the gallery is rarely crowded. While you may encounter a few photography fans or even a random Hotel Commonwealth guest, you are just as likely to have the place all to yourself. I like to stop by with art-loving friends around midafternoon on a Saturday, and then head downstairs to Island Creek Oyster Bar for a glass of wine and some Massachusetts bivalves.

✌ essentials

502c Commonwealth Avenue, Boston, MA 02215

(617) 267-8929

panopticongallery.com
hotelcommonwealth.com

$ Free

Tuesday–Saturday, 10 a.m.–5:30 p.m.

T: Green Line, B, C, or D train, to Kenmore

peaceful place 95

PAUL REVERE MALL

North End, Boston (MAP THREE)

CATEGORY ⌣ historic sites ⭐

*M*ention the Paul Revere Mall to me and, in my mind, I hear the calming sounds of a fountain, church bells, voices speaking Italian, and dominoes clicking together on a warm afternoon. Flanked on one end by the Old North Church and on the other by St. Stephen's across Hanover Street, the location is, to me, the heart of Boston's North End.

Though the dominant mall feature is Cyrus Edwin Dallin's iconic statute of Paul Revere astride his horse, I've always been more captivated by the stories told on the 13 bronze plaques that line the walls of what locals call the *prado*, a Spanish word sometimes translated to "meadow" in English. A trip here is like meandering through a brief history of the North End, from Ann Pollard who arrived here in 1630 as a child of 10, to Benjamin Franklin who lived here as a boy, to the many heroes of World War I.

(Dallin, by the way, created two other world-famous works: *Appeal to the Great Spirit*, which stands at the front entrance of Boston's Museum of Fine Arts, and the *Angel Moroni*, which stands atop the landmark Mormon church, the Salt Lake Temple, in Utah.)

Tree-shaded benches provide perfect spots to daydream as you watch people amble by—and it's a varied, fascinating group, including Italian grandmothers sharing a bit of gossip, teenagers horsing around, and tourists resolutely following the Freedom Trail.

⌣ **essentials**

▣	Hanover Street between Tileston and Charter streets, Boston, MA 02109
✆ n/a	🌐 paul-revere-heritage.com/landmarks.html $ Free
�🕐 Daily, sunrise–sunset	T: Orange Line or Green Line to Haymarket

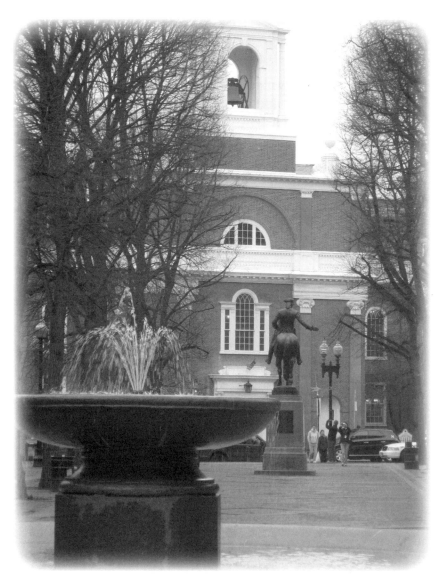

St. Stephen's Church (in the background) and Paul Revere's statue

peaceful place 96

PETER FANEUIL HOUSE GARDEN

Beacon Hill, Boston (MAP TWO)

CATEGORY ᴗ̈ urban surprises ✪ ✪ ✪

While Beacon Hill is famous for its hidden gardens, there's only one time a year that you can view them: that day in mid-May when the Beacon Hill Garden Club hosts its annual tour. However, if you'd like to get a hint of the tranquility to be found in one of those tiny oases, you can satisfy that desire with a visit to the Peter Faneuil House Garden, located next to a historic building that was once a school and has been renovated for modern-day affordable housing.

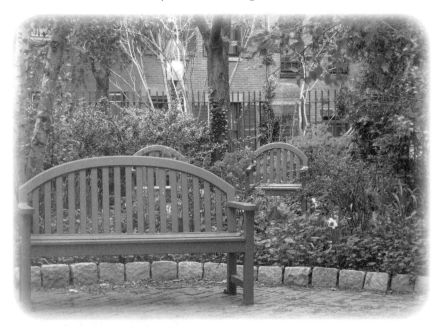

Welcoming benches in a secluded garden

When you walk through the park's iron gate, you enter a world of brick and greenery. Flowering crab apple trees, daffodils, and bright crimson azaleas greet you in the spring. In summer, it's delightful to pause on one of the red benches and savor the shade offered by the birch trees. With a light dusting of snow, the garden feels like a secret winter sanctuary.

Though the garden lies only a brief walk from the hustle and bustle around Park Street, it's on the quieter side of Beacon Hill. Nonresidents rarely venture to this area, making it a perfect stop for someone in need of a little solitude.

But back to that garden tour available only once a year: the Beacon Hill Garden Club also maintains the Faneuil House Garden, and the organization earmarks part of the proceeds from that annual event to care for this special place.

essentials

30 South Russell Street, Boston, MA 02114

n/a

Visit beaconhillgardenclub.org for more on the Beacon Hill Garden Club's annual event.

$ Free

Daily, sunrise–sunset

T: Red Line to Charles/MGH; Green Line, any train, to Park

peaceful place 97

PIERS PARK

East Boston (MAP SEVEN)
CATEGORY ⌣ scenic vistas ✪ ✪

*E*ast Boston's location on the inner harbor offers panoramic views of the downtown Boston skyline, including such historic sites as Old North Church and the Custom House. But until Piers Park was built, in 1995, on the site of an abandoned wharf, there was no good place to relax and appreciate that scenery.

Though extremely popular with East Boston locals, the 6.5-acre park seems to be little known to Bostonians from other neighborhoods, which is a shame. The lush green lawn invites you to spread out a picnic, strike a few yoga asanas, or play a relaxed game of

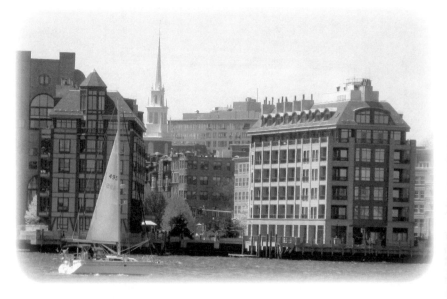

Old North Church, with its famous steeple, as seen from Piers Park

catch. Children love frolicking on the grass or at the well-appointed playground. Benches welcome you to read, share a quiet conversation, or simply admire the views.

When it's time for a leisurely stroll, follow the 600-foot pedestrian walkway to the water's edge. There are six pavilions along the way, where you'll find both shade and descriptive panels that celebrate the history, culture, and ethnic diversity of East Boston.

While weekday hours are the most tranquil, the sunsets over the city can be quite dramatic, and this setting offers a great way to refresh your spirits at the end of a busy day. Get off at the Maverick T station, pick up some picnic fixings or takeout from one of the restaurants or shops in Maverick Square, and then walk the couple of blocks to the park entrance and prepare to be dazzled.

❧ essentials

⊟ 95 Marginal Street between Clyde and Haynes streets, Boston, MA 02128

☎ (617) 568-5000

🌐 massport.com/port-of-boston
bostonharborwalk.com/placestogo (Click on "East Boston" on the display map, and then "Piers Park" in the pop-up menu.)

$ Free

🕐 **Spring–summer:** Daily, 6 a.m.–11:30 p.m. **Fall–winter:** Daily, sunrise–sunset

🚇 **T:** Blue Line to Maverick

peaceful place 98

PORTSMOUTH EXCURSION

Portsmouth, NH (MAP TEN)

CATEGORY ↻ day trips & overnights ✪

*B*arely a 90-minute drive north of Boston, even with heavy traffic, Portsmouth is New Hampshire's only city by the sea—though one could argue that it feels much more like a charming little town. The streets and parks invite strolling; locals own most of the restaurants, shops, and galleries; and concerts, theater, and other events provide a respectable cultural scene.

Those looking for some quiet outdoor fun will find plenty to love as well. A bike ride around the NH 1B loop takes you out of Portsmouth, along the tidal river, and into quaint New Castle. There you can visit the historic Wentworth by the Sea hotel and enjoy a spa treatment or, in summer, have lunch at the hotel's Latitudes Waterfront, overlooking the marina at Little Harbor.

From Portsmouth, a longer bicycle ride—or picturesque drive, if you prefer—heads back south on NH 1A, along the coast, to North Hampton. Though on summer weekends the road gets a bit hectic, the shoreline offers plenty of rocky nooks and crannies where you can stop and find a spot to see and hear nothing but pounding surf.

For a more mellow experience, try kayaking up Sagamore Creek. I first discovered this usually tranquil tidal waterway when my parents moved to Portsmouth in the early 1990s. If you have your own craft, you can launch it at Witch Cove Marina for a charge of $20. Or you can rent a single or double boat from Portsmouth Kayak Adventures (PKA). For the ultimate in serenity, try one of their full-moon paddling excursions. PKA also rents out bicycles by the day or half day.

Those looking for peaceful fine dining with an emphasis on local ingredients will enjoy Black Trumpet Bistro, in the Portsmouth Historic District. For a casual meal, and the ultimate lobster experience, venture a little farther up the coast to Chauncey Creek at Kittery Point in Maine, where you sit on bright-colored picnic tables just above water level. At Chauncey Creek, you're welcome to bring your own wine, cocktails, appetizers, and salads—some people even bring tablecloths and flowers! If you're considering an overnight stay, most rooms at the Wentworth have water views. Or stay in town at the Victorian-style Sise Inn.

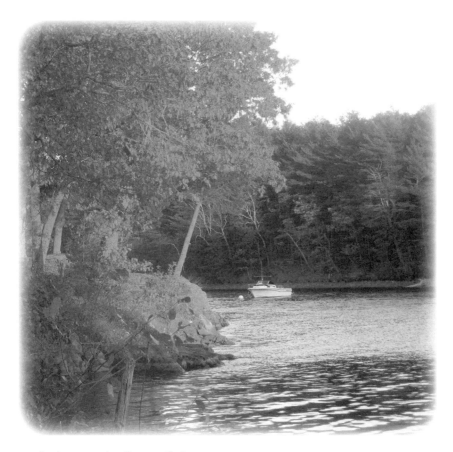

Lovely contours along Sagamore Creek

⌣ essentials

[=•]   **Wentworth by the Sea, a Marriott Hotel and Spa:** 588 Wentworth Road,
New Castle, NH 03854
Portsmouth Kayak Adventures: 185 Wentworth Road, Portsmouth, NH 03801
Portsmouth Bike Rentals: 91 Marcy Street, Portsmouth, NH 03801
Black Trumpet Bistro: 29 Ceres Street, Portsmouth, NH 03801
Chauncey Creek Lobster Pier: 16 Chauncey Creek Road, Kittery Point, ME 03905
Sise Inn: 40 Court Street, Portsmouth, NH 03801

(*)   **Wentworth by the Sea, a Marriott Hotel and Spa:** (603) 422-7322; **Portsmouth Kayak Adventures:** (603) 559-1000; **Portsmouth Bike Rentals:** (603) 431-1266; **Black Trumpet Bistro:** (603) 431-0887; **Chauncey Creek Lobster Pier:** (207) 439-1030; **Sise Inn:** (603) 433-1200

(*)   wentworth.com
portsmouthkayak.com
portsmouthbikerentals.com
blacktrumpetbistro.com
chaunceycreek.com
siseinn.com

$ **Wentworth by the Sea, a Marriott Hotel and Spa:** $219–$999 per night; **Portsmouth Kayak Adventures:** $35–$84; **Portsmouth Bike Rentals:** $25–$40; **Black Trumpet Bistro:** $6–$31; **Chauncey Creek Lobster Pier:** $4–market price; **Sise Inn:** $119–$299 per night

(*)   **Portsmouth Kayak Adventures** and **Portsmouth Bike Rentals:** May–October. **Black Trumpet Bistro:** Daily, from 5:30 p.m. **Chauncey Creek Lobster Pier:** Mother's Day–Labor Day: Daily, 11 a.m.–8 p.m. After Labor Day–Columbus Day: Tuesday–Sunday, 11 a.m.–7 p.m.

   n/a

peaceful place 99

PROVINCETOWN EXCURSION

Cape Cod, MA (MAP ELEVEN)

CATEGORY ⌣: day trips & overnights ⭐

*D*espite what you might remember from history class, the Pilgrims' first landfall in the New World was not at Plymouth Rock but rather at the north tip of Cape

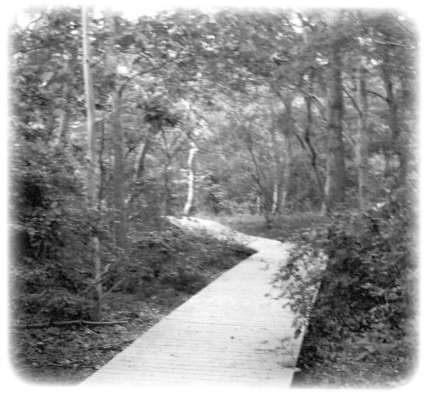

photographed by Tony Siracusa

A boardwalk through the Beech Forest

Cod, where Provincetown sits today. Unlike more recent visitors, the Pilgrims found the area not to their liking and moved on to a more sheltered spot on Massachusetts Bay.

Ironically, Provincetown's very position on an exposed, narrow strip of land between two large bodies of water is what gives the light there the magical characteristics so beloved by artists, photographers, and nature lovers. Though summer is when most people visit, I prefer Provincetown during its quieter fall season. The angle of the sun combined with the colors of trees and scrub means that land and seascapes are at their most striking.

You'll want to spend some time wandering through town. A growing number of shops, galleries, and restaurants here stay open all year now, as late fall, winter, and early spring have become popular times to visit. The Cape Cod National Seashore offers more than 7 miles of paved trails for walking or bicycling. (You can rent bikes in town.) Herring Cove, one of the few beaches on the East Coast that faces west—because of the cape's curving "arm"—is a wonderful spot to catch the sunset.

For a less-expected taste of the Cape's natural beauty, visit my favorite place here, the Beech Forest. This is the "Provincelands" that Pulitzer Prize–winning poet Mary Oliver writes about, with its woodlands, marshes, and freshwater ponds. And walking here is like slipping into one of her poems. Oliver lives in Provincetown, and her words give this setting shape in so many of her books. You'll sense a mixture of salt and pine in the air here. In the distance, you can hear the roar of the open Atlantic. Chickadees and titmice may swoop down to see if you've brought them any birdseed. Walk quietly and you may even see a deer.

The entrance to Beech Forest lies on the left, 0.5 mile up Race Point Road from U.S. 6. The 0.75-mile pond loop skirts around the edge of two freshwater ponds; the 0.25-mile extension loop takes you a little deeper into the woods. Together, they require about an hour to traverse. (Be sure to wear sturdy, comfortable shoes, and bring bug spray.)

If you don't mind a lot of driving—about $2^{1}/_{2}$ hours each way—Provincetown can be a day trip. But to inspire a quieter mood, make it at least one overnight. I've found the Fairbanks Inn in the center of town to be comfortable, friendly, and reasonably priced. For dining, friends who are locals recommend the Mews, Fanizzi's, or Napi's.

✌ essentials

☰ Provincetown, MA, is 115 miles southeast of Boston.
Cape Cod National Seashore: 99 Marconi Site Road, Wellfleet, MA 02667
Fairbanks Inn: 90 Bradford Street, Provincetown, MA 02657
Mews: 429 Commercial Street, Provincetown, MA 02657
Fanizzi's: 539 Commercial Street, Provincetown, MA 02657
Napi's: 7 Freeman Street, Provincetown, MA 02657

☏ **Cape Cod National Seashore:** (508) 771-2144; **Fairbanks Inn:** (800) 324-7265; **Mews:**
(508) 487-1500; **Fanizzi's:** (508) 487-1964; **Napi's:** (800) 571-6274

🌐 **Provincetown information:** provincetown.com
Cape Cod National Seashore: nps.gov/caco
Fairbanks Inn: fairbanksinn.com
Mews: mews.com
Fanizzi's: fanizzisrestaurant.com
Napi's: napis-restaurant.com

$ **Cape Cod National Seashore beaches** (late June–early September when lifeguards
are on duty, and Saturday–Sunday and holidays Memorial Day–September): vehicles:
$15 per day; pedestrians and bicyclists: $3 per day; annual pass: $45. **Fairbanks Inn:**
$100–$325 per night; **Mews:** $19–$33; **Fanizzi's:** $7–$26; **Napi's:** $5–$34

🕐 **Cape Cod National Seashore:** Beaches and trails: Daily, year-round, but may be
closed due to weather. Parking lots: Daily, 6 a.m.–midnight. **Mews:** Daily, from 6 p.m.
Fanizzi's: Daily, 11:30 a.m.–4 p.m. and 4:30 p.m.–close. Brunch: Sunday, 10 a.m.–2 p.m.
Closed Thanksgiving and December 25. **Napi's:** May–September: Daily, from 5 p.m.
October–April: Lunch: Daily, from 11:30 a.m. Dinner: Daily, from 5 p.m.

🚌 In fall and winter, Plymouth & Brockton Street Railway Co., in business since 1888,
offers bus service twice daily between Boston and Provincetown. (Trips are more
frequent in spring and summer.) The trip takes a little more than 3 hours. Check the
schedule at **p-b.com.** For additional information on bus transportation and seasonal
ferry service from Boston to Provincetown, visit **nps.gov/caco/planyourvisit/
publictransportation.htm** and/or **smartguide.org.**

peaceful place 100

PRUDENTIAL CENTER SOUTH GARDEN

Back Bay, Boston (MAP ONE)

CATEGORY ⌣: urban surprises ✪ ✪

*I*nside the Prudential Center Mall, shoppers, office workers, and convention-goers hurry about their business. But when you step through one of the doors that opens into the South Garden, you feel as though you're entering another world. With its groves of trees and abundant shrubs, grasses, and perennials, including roses, astilbe, and rudbeckia, the 1.3-acre open-air plaza offers a quiet refuge.

The large fountain, shaped like a black disk set on a squat oblong pedestal, drowns out the city noises beyond. The water feature that's part of the large sculpture in the southwest corner creates the illusion that the people sitting in that area are floating on water. The tables at the west entrance offer a comfortable spot to settle with takeout food, read, or just enjoy the sun and the scenery. Kids can't seem to resist using the lush green lawn for cartwheels and somersaults, and even adults seem to enjoy sitting there.

In summer, the garden is sometimes used for concerts and films. While it can get a little crowded then and at lunchtime, most times you can find a shady nook where you can just relax and get away from it all.

☌ essentials

🖃 800 Boylston Street, Boston, MA 02199   📞 (617) 236-2300

🌐 prudentialcenter.com/explore/about.php

$ Free   🕐 **Spring–fall:** Daily, 8 a.m.–8 p.m., depending on weather

🚍 **T:** Green Line E to Prudential Center

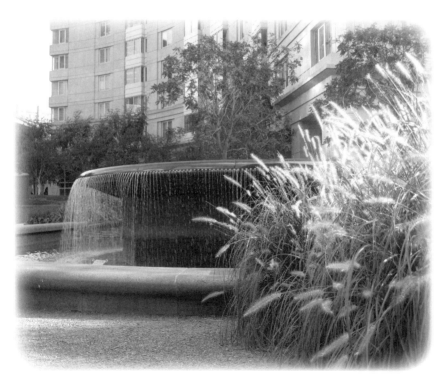

An oasis in the middle of a mall

peaceful place 101

RADCLIFFE INSTITUTE FOR ADVANCED STUDY, SUNKEN GARDEN

Cambridge, MA (MAP SIX)

CATEGORY ⌣ parks & gardens ✪ ✪

*C*ould there be a more appropriate location for an Eden-like oasis than in Cambridge where Garden Street meets Appian Way? Here at the Sunken Garden, just off the Radcliffe Quadrangle, theatrical performances are given, concerts and poetry readings are held, and even wedding vows are made. Yet most days, the space just provides a lovely escape, where you can pretend to be a college student immersing yourself in a book or soaking up some sun.

My favorite route into the Sunken Garden is from the side closest to Brattle Street. From this approach, the fountain area, with its bed of black river rocks and low stone wall, seems to draw you in, welcoming you to linger on one of the six memorial benches.

If you find the main garden too full of earnest young scholars for your taste, follow the narrow path that leads to the large beech tree at the Garden Street edge. Here, you'll find a lovely shade garden, overflowing with Epimedium, false Solomon's seal, Fothergilla, and ferns. There are benches here, too, though they rarely seem to be occupied. Happily, the fountain is close enough to muffle the street sounds, promising to lull you into a well-deserved repose.

essentials

☰ Garden Street and Appian Way, Cambridge, MA 02138

☎ n/a

🌐 Visit radcliffe.edu for information on the institute.

$ Free

🕐 Daily, sunrise–sunset

🚌 **T:** Red Line to Harvard

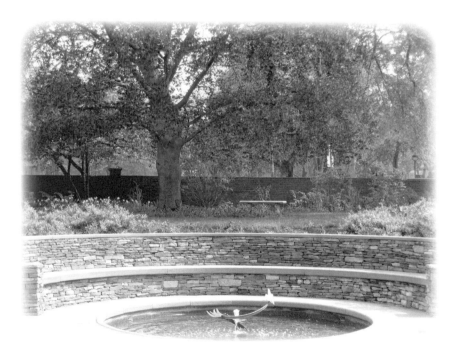

Your refuge on a busy campus

peaceful place 102

RAVEN USED BOOKS

Back Bay, Boston (MAP ONE)

CATEGORY ⌣ shops & services ✪ ✪

*J*oyce, Nabokov, Wolfe, Auden. Sounds like a class I took in college. Actually, those are the authors whose titles were displayed on outdoor shelves the first time I stopped by Raven Used Books. Also outside, you can still count on a comfortable bench on the small patio to offer refuge from the crowds on Newbury Street.

This Raven location remains a small store, but it is big on atmosphere. Inside, cool jazz plays on the sound system, and you can browse to your heart's content. The shop is home to one of the most impressive collections of used books in the city. Hard-to-find titles, too, await in almost perfect condition. The subject matter is definitely a little more highbrow than your average used-bookstore inventory. Though there's a solid fiction section, it's oriented more toward the classics than, say, Tom Clancy best sellers. While I'm most impressed by the superb selection of design, art, and architecture books, the wide range of titles in philosophy, history, anthropology, religion, and poetry is pleasing as well. Raven is also a good place to look for children's books.

Prices are quite reasonable, considering the quality: most books cost no more than half the original cover price. According to its website, Raven (which has a bigger store in Harvard Square) adds more than 1,000 titles a week, so there's always fresh stock on the shelves. I can't vouch that some 1,000 new titles come in weekly, but I do know from experience that, if you see something you want, you better get it because it's likely to be gone by your next visit.

↭ essentials

✉ 263 Newbury Street, Boston, MA 02116   ✆ (617) 578-9000

🌐 ravencambridge.com

$ Free, except for purchases; **books:** typically at least 50% off the original cover price

🕐 Monday–Saturday, 10 a.m.–9 p.m.; Sunday, 11 a.m.–8 p.m.

🚆 **T:** Green Line, B, C, or D train, to Hynes Auditorium

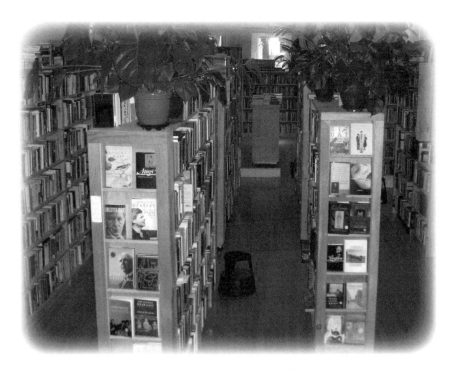

A dazzling selection of books in the arts, history, classics, and philosophy

peaceful place 103

RESTAURANT DANTE

East Cambridge, MA (MAP SEVEN)

CATEGORY ◡ quiet tables ✪

*W*hen the street that separates the Royal Sonesta Hotel Boston from the Charles River was transformed from a bustling four-lane highway to a quiet, 20-foot-wide parkway, the Sonesta was able to offer an amenity that can't be found anywhere else along the river: peaceful, waterfront patio dining, with spectacular views of Beacon Hill and the Back Bay across the water.

Restaurant Dante, which chef Dante de Magistris has operated here with his brothers Filippo and Damian since 2006, is more than worthy of this location. A dish of his

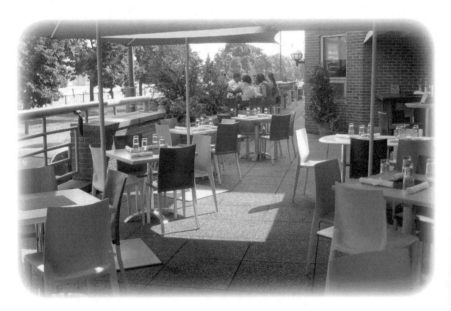

Outdoor dining with a river view

homemade pasta—particularly the saffron-laced *strozzapreti* with clams, calamari, rock shrimp, and zucchini—and a glass of, perhaps, Matteo Correggia Arneis make you feel as though you've been transported to a serene seaside town in Italy.

While you can't make reservations for the patio, early weeknights are usually a good bet for landing a table alfresco. The accommodating staff is also pretty flexible as to what constitutes suitable weather for outdoor service. I was there on a night when showers were passing through, yet a couple who requested a patio table was cheerfully seated there.

And no worries if you do sit inside: The large windows give those tables a pleasant view as well. And here I'll let out one of the city's best-kept secrets: Dante's patio is a great place to catch the Fourth of July fireworks display bursting forth on the other side of the river.

⌣: essentials

Royal Sonesta Hotel Boston, 40 Edwin H. Land Boulevard, Cambridge, MA 02142

(617) 497-4200

restaurantdante.com

$ Lunch: $10–$24; **Dinner:** $16–$38

Year-round: Monday–Thursday, 5:30–10 p.m.; Friday–Saturday, 5:30–11 p.m.; Sunday, 5–9 p.m. **Bar:** 2:30 p.m.–close. **May–September:** Monday–Friday, 11:30 a.m.– 2:30 p.m.

T: Green Line to Science Park

peaceful place 104

RICKY'S FLOWER MARKET

Somerville, MA (MAP SEVEN)

CATEGORY ↝ shops & services ✪

*I*n Paris, there's the Marché aux Fleurs; in Rome, the Campo dei Fiori; in the Boston area, there's Ricky's Flower Market in Somerville. Located on the site of a former gas station, at the crossroads of a busy intersection, Ricky's is like a fragrant green oasis in the midst of a chaotic urban landscape.

As you wander the narrow pathways between the tables bedecked with plants of every description, from dwarf fruit trees to grasses, ferns to ornamental conifers, and flowers to herbs, you'll feel as though the noise of the traffic around you is melting away in a swirl of scent and color.

While Ricky's is a destination for the pumpkins, dried arrangements, and evergreens necessary for fall and winter celebrations, it's in its glory in late spring, when the weather softens enough to be safe for tender perennials and annuals. Even if you just come away with a few pansies for an outside planter or a pot of basil for your windowsill, you'll feel refreshed, as though you've just spent a few moments in the Garden of Eden.

↝ essentials

⊟ 238 Washington Street, Somerville, MA 02143

☎ (617) 628-7569   ⊕ rickysflowermarket.com $ Free

🕐 **Mid-March–late December:** Monday–Saturday, 9 a.m.–7 p.m.; Sunday, 9 a.m.–6 p.m.

🚌 T: Orange Line to Sullivan Square or Red Line to Central Square, and then Bus 91 to Union Square

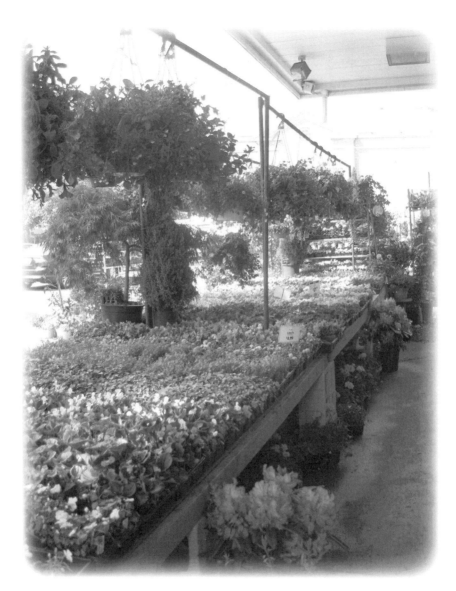

A mecca for gardeners and flower lovers

peaceful place 105

RIVERWAY

The Fenway, Boston (MAP FIVE: SEE 105; MAP EIGHT: SEE 105A AND 105B)

CATEGORY ⌣ parks & gardens ⭐

O n most Boston maps, the Riverway appears as a busy roadway. In reality, it's also the polar opposite—a linear ribbon of tranquility. Part of Frederick Law Olmsted's Emerald Necklace, the Riverway stretches for 34 acres, a little less than a mile in distance, along the Boston–Brookline border, from Park Drive to MA 9.

While cars rush along the Boston edge, people on foot and bicycles move alongside the Muddy River on circa 1890 bridle and walking paths set considerably below street

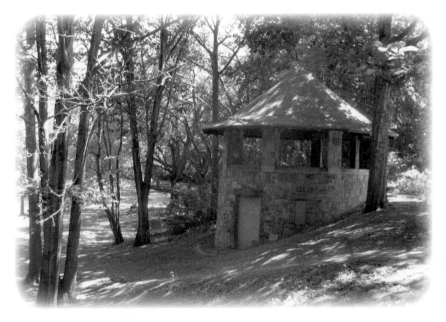

The stone gazebo at the Chapel Street Bridge

level. This is a summertime peaceful place, when the leaf canopy on the statuesque oaks screens out the traffic noise and the blazing sun, creating a serene oasis. Every now and then, you walk beneath a picturesque old stone bridge, and strategically placed benches along the way lure you for relaxation and contemplation. The landscape and hills are not natural but were created to provide a beautiful, healthful environment for the enjoyment of city residents. (In fact, the Muddy River is not natural either, as Olmsted had the original waterway dredged to create a winding stream that emptied into the Charles.)

Technically, the Brookline side of the path is considered a bikeway, while the Boston side is for pedestrians, but I think the former is quieter—even though in places it runs along the Green Line tracks—and it provides a better view of the river. For a round-trip excursion, head out on one side and return on the other.

If you have the time, and don't mind crossing a few busy intersections, you can continue on through Olmsted Park all the way to Jamaica Pond. If you do, be sure to pause by the two small secluded ponds you'll pass along the way, Willow Pond and Ward's Pond. Between the two is the site of an abandoned ice-skating rink that, to the delight of local butterflies, has now become a wildflower meadow.

essentials

🖃	Emerald Necklace, from Park Drive to MA 9, Boston, MA 02215 and Brookline, MA 02245 and 02446
☎	(617) 522-2700
🌐	emeraldnecklace.org/parks/riverway
$	Free
🕐	Daily, 7 a.m.–11:30 p.m.
🚗	**T:** Green Line, D train, to Fenway

peaceful place 106

ROSE ART MUSEUM

Waltham, MA (MAP NINE)

CATEGORY ⌣ museums & galleries ✪ ✪

*I*n early 2009, the president of Brandeis University made a stunning announcement: the university had decided to shut down the Rose Art Museum and sell its 7,500 works of art. Those pieces were widely considered to be the largest, preeminent collection of modern and contemporary art amassed anywhere in New England.

Fortunately for those with a passion for great art—and for the inviting places in which to contemplate it—this did not come to pass. Less than 3 years later, the Rose celebrated its 50th anniversary in a newly revitalized space, with the guarantee that neither the museum nor its collection was in jeopardy.

Though the art on display always discharges plenty of psychic energy, I find a visit to the Rose to be a calming, refreshing experience. Exhibitions change once or twice a year,

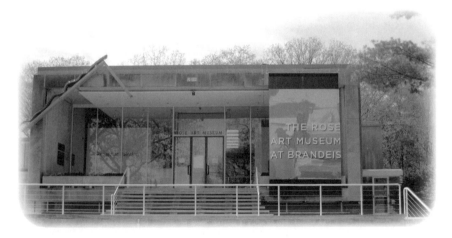

Exterior of the museum, a half-hour's drive west of Boston

usually at the beginning of a semester. Some focus solely on works from the permanent collection, which includes Willem de Kooning, Jasper Johns, Roy Lichtenstein, Hans Hofmann, Ellsworth Kelly, and Helen Frankenthaler. Other shows may incorporate works borrowed from other institutions or private collectors.

Despite the quality of the art, the Rose is rarely crowded. The open, airy galleries invite leisurely exploration, and plenty of benches allow you to pause and ponder what you've seen. Students from the university's art program often can be found here seeking inspiration. That young person sketching in the corner may be a future Andy Warhol or Judy Chicago.

ᗢ essentials

✉	415 South Street, Waltham, MA 02453
☎	(781) 736-3434
🌐	brandeis.edu/rose
$	Free
🕐	Tuesday–Sunday, noon–5 p.m.
🚃	**T:** Commuter Rail, Fitchburg Line/South Acton Line, to Brandeis/Roberts

peaceful place 107

SACRED SPACE, NORTHEASTERN UNIVERSITY

The Fenway, Boston (MAP FIVE)

CATEGORY ↙ spiritual enclaves ✪ ✪ ✪

*I*n 1996, fire destroyed the chapel at Northeastern University. When it came time to rebuild, the school chose instead to create a setting that would celebrate its spiritual diversity: The Sacred Space.

As you enter through the western entrance, you'll find an ablution area, with a low stainless steel sink to accommodate ritual foot washing. Often you're greeted by the sound of chanting or the low murmuring of prayer coming from one of the personal contemplation spaces beyond.

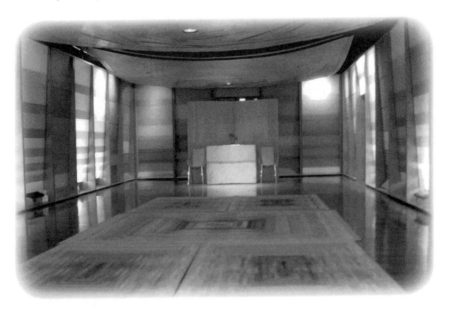

Serenity at the Sacred Space

The Sacred Space is located to the left of the entrance. At what would be the narthex, if this were a church, you're welcome to pick up a meditation cushion, yoga mat, or pillow if you desire. Inside, the light is dim, there's the hushed sound of white noise, and the entire room seems bathed in a gentle glow. Immediately to your left is a simple sculpture where the phrase "May peace prevail on earth" is written in 12 languages, including sign language and, somewhat fancifully, animal tracks!

On the Northeastern website, the Sacred Space is described as offering "an atmosphere of peace, a sense of the holy and a refuge for prayer, contemplation or meditation." I can't imagine a more accurate portrayal of this simple, yet deeply spiritual place.

essentials

203 Ell Hall, 360 Huntington Avenue, Boston, MA 02115

(617) 373-2728

northeastern.edu/spirituallife/space.html

Free

During fall and winter semesters: Monday–Saturday, 9 a.m.–10 p.m.; Sunday and most holidays, 11 a.m.–10 p.m. **Summer hours:** Monday–Friday, 9 a.m.–9 p.m.; Saturday, 9 a.m.–7 p.m. Closed Memorial Day; July 4; Thanksgiving weekend (Wednesday evening–Saturday); and December 23–the first Monday in January. Hours vary during the first week in May.

T: Green Line, E train, to Northeastern University

peaceful place 108

SEAPORT PARKS

Seaport District, Boston (MAP FOUR)

CATEGORY ↙ parks & gardens ✪

*T*hough separated only by the southbound lane of D Street, the South Boston Maritime Park and the Eastport Park couldn't be more different. The former, owned by the Massachusetts Port Authority, is an active public space. The other, under management of a division of Fidelity Investments, is a more serene sculpture garden.

Both parks, however, possess an abundance of charm. Maritime Park has a clam shack–inspired café, large pergolas, fog fountain (much beloved by the younger set), tide lights that respond to the daily tidal fluctuations, and numerous marine-themed granite features—all in little over an acre of space. The gently sloped lawn enables one to enjoy water views, regardless of the tide level. (Don't miss Carlos Dorrien's *Gateway* sculpture, with its fanciful depictions of fish, sea life, and the ocean floor.)

Those seeking a bit of shade and serenity might consider an escape to the park's opposite side, where there's a beautifully landscaped bosk—a wooded area surrounded by abundant foliage. Or you just may want to wander across D Street, where the enticing 1.6-acre Eastport Park offers a number of secluded tree-lined nooks, surrounded by banks of flowers and shrubs.

Eastport, too, has a nautical theme, but it's cozier and quieter. The front wild garden, overflowing with grasses and perennials, was designed to be reminiscent of something you'd find on the coast of Maine. At the rear, eight large London plane trees muffle the noise from Congress Street. Throughout, plantings provide a respite from the sun, tempting you to pause on the charming fish benches and savor the harbor's sounds and smells. Or you may be inspired to go beachcombing along the winding paths in search of stone or metal creatures, such as David Phillips's whimsical frogs, shrimp, and hermit crabs.

Strategically placed rocks with divots that hold rainwater conjure up visions of tide-pools. *Wind Traveler,* the sea breeze–powered kinetic sculpture by Susumu Shingu, not only resembles a multi-masted schooner, but it also undergoes annual maintenance at a yacht yard in Salem to keep its bearings and sails shipshape! Before you leave, be sure to look for Wendy Ross's sculpture, *Leviathan,* a 100-foot-long piece that appears to slither down the grand staircase at the nearby World Trade Center West.

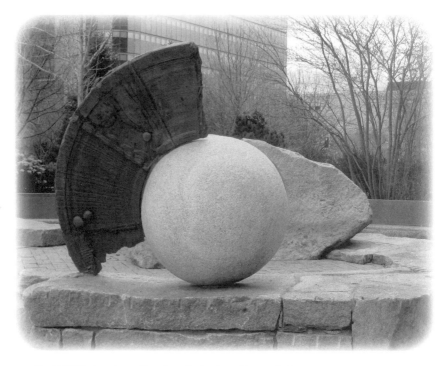

David Phillips's sculpture Chords: *a focal point at Eastport Park*

✌ essentials

⌨   Seaport Avenue and Northern Avenue at D Street, Boston, MA 02210

☏   (617) 482-1722

🌐   bostonharborwalk.com/placestogo (Click on "South Boston," and then on "Eastport Park" or "South Boston Maritime Park" on the drop-down menu. For viewing pleasure, be sure to click on the individual photos of the sculptures on each of these specific sites.)

$ Free

🕐   Daily, sunrise–sunset

🚌   **T:** Silver Line to World Trade Center

peaceful place 109

SOUTHWEST CORRIDOR PARK

South End, Boston (MAP FOUR)

CATEGORY ↙ enchanting walks ✪ ✪

oston's Southwest Corridor Park stretches 4.7 miles, from Copley Square to Forest Hills. Some 25 minigarden spaces dot the 10-block South End section, between Huntington and Columbus avenues. While the city owns the land, volunteers from the Southwest Corridor Park Conservancy design and maintain the gardens.

I like to think of this as a refreshing walk bookended by poems and stories. "Drum," a poem by Sharon Cox Howell, and "I Know My Robe Gonna Fit Me Well," a story by Peter Rodman, are engraved on granite monuments just beyond the western boundary, near the Massachusetts Avenue T station. "Counterpoint," a story by Jane Barnes, and "If My Boundary Stops Here," a poem by Ruth Whitman, are at the eastern end across Dartmouth Street from Back Bay Station.* Somehow, I feel that taking a moment to read at least one of these at the beginning or end of my walks here makes the journey seem even more special.

Though it's best when the gardens are blooming, visits to this park are a pleasure in every season. In spring, the flowering crab apple trees provide a canopy of pink and white. On wintry days, snow outlines the stark silhouettes of shrubs and trees. At the western end, a butterfly garden supports the life cycle of six species of butterflies, including monarchs, red admirals, and black swallowtails. Near the eastern end, a newly restored garden provides a relaxing place to linger beneath a pair of mature dogwood trees—appropriately enough, as it overlooks the local dog park.

You likely will hear occasional train whistles—both the MBTA's Orange Line and Amtrak trains are passing beneath your feet. That is because some park areas are planted on decks above the train tracks. However, you will feel sheltered from most of the city's sounds. If you have time, a leisurely side trip down Bradford Park, Holyoke Street, and

West Canton Street offers a look at some of the residential parks that give this part of the South End its distinctive character. Most are nicely landscaped, with cast-iron fencing and a central fountain.

Note: Seven other stories and poems, part of the Boston Contemporary Writers Program, can be found near Orange Line stations from Tufts Medical Center along the rest of the Southwest Corridor to Forest Hills.

✓ essentials

📧 Between St. Botolph Street and Columbus Avenue, from Centre Street to Yarmouth Street, and between Lamartine and Amory streets, from Centre Street to Green Street, to MA 203, Boston, MA 02119, 02118, 02116, 02120, and 02130

☎ (617) 727-0057

🌐 swcpc.org/swcpmap.htm
mass.gov/dcr/parks/metroboston/southwestCorr.htm
For images of the story/poem stones, visit
nuweb.neu.edu/psullivan/massaveone.html
and nuweb.neu.edu/psullivan/backbaystationone.html

$ Free

🕐 Open 24/7

🚇 T: Orange Line to Back Bay or Massachusetts Avenue stations

peaceful place 110

SOWA DISTRICT
South End, Boston (MAP FOUR)
CATEGORY ⌣ shops & services ✪

*A*s rents on Newbury Street skyrocketed and the cachet of the South End grew, galleries and artists began flocking to a section of that neighborhood now affectionately known as SoWa, in honor of its location south of Washington Street.

The SoWa Artists Guild, a series of former warehouse buildings at 450–460 Harrison Avenue, is home to 15 galleries and more than 50 artist studios. In response, other art- and design-related businesses have taken up residence there as well. Though the building hums with activity on the first Friday of the month when artists open their studios to showcase their recent work, many artists also quietly welcome visitors during off hours, especially by appointment.

Just down the street is the equally fascinating—and frequently quite tranquil—Boston Sculptors Gallery, an artists' cooperative and one of the only places in Boston where contemporary sculpture is always on display. Of course, on those occasions when the current exhibit features loud video and blinking lights, you may need to search for serenity elsewhere.

If you're just as interested in reading about art as looking at it, a visit to Ars Libri is a must. Here, you can browse through one of the largest selections of rare and out-of-print art-related books anywhere. But be advised: That alluring scent of old bindings and paper might tempt you to purchase a treasure for your own library.

The SoWa Open Market and SoWa Vintage Market, with their authentic artisan's bazaar atmosphere, make this neighborhood the place to see and be seen on Sundays in season. Know that satisfying feeling of peace that comes with doing something fascinating and fun? This is the place to get it. The crowds thin out a bit toward the end of the day, so if you don't mind the possibility of missing out on a bargain or treasure (and aren't worried about the food trucks running out of your favorite ethnic treat), stop by then. Otherwise, keep in mind the quiet little garden space near the Boston Sculptors Gallery. It offers an oasis of calm, as you linger over that tasty Asian snack.

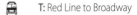 essentials

SoWa Artists Guild: 450 Harrison Avenue, Boston, MA 02118
Boston Sculptors Gallery: 486 Harrison Avenue, Boston, MA 02118
Ars Libri Ltd.: 500 Harrison Avenue, Boston, MA 02118
SoWa Open Market: 460 Harrison Avenue, Boston, MA 02118
SoWa Vintage Market: 460c Harrison Avenue, Boston, MA 02118

SoWa Artists Guild: Visit website (see below) and click on "Directory" for individual artists' phone numbers; **Boston Sculptors Gallery:** (617) 482-7781; **Ars Libri Ltd.:** (617) 357-5212; **SoWa Open Market:** (800) 403-8305

sowaartistsguild.com
bostonsculptors.com
arslibri.com
sowaopenmarket.com
sowavintagemarket.com

$ Free, except for purchases

SoWa Artists Guild: Monday–Friday, 9 a.m.–7 p.m.; Saturday–Sunday, 11 a.m.–5 p.m.; First Friday of each month: 5–9 p.m.
Boston Sculptors Gallery: Wednesday–Sunday, noon–6 p.m.; closed January 1, Thanksgiving, and December 25
Ars Libri Ltd.: Monday–Friday, 9 a.m.–6 p.m.; Saturday, 11 a.m.–5 p.m.; closed Saturdays in August
SoWa Open Market: May–October: Sunday, 10 a.m.–4 p.m.
SoWa Vintage Market: Sunday, 10 a.m.–4 p.m.

T: Red Line to Broadway

peaceful place 111

SWAN BOATS OF BOSTON

Public Garden, Boston (MAP ONE)

CATEGORY 🏞 parks & gardens ✪

It may seem strange to find one of Boston's most famous tourist attractions listed in *Peaceful Places*. In truth, the crowds of schoolchildren who visit on weekdays in the spring and the tourists who flock here in the summer can make this spot anything but tranquil. Yet there's something both charming and unexpectedly calming about gliding through the water in a foot-propelled watercraft shaped like a swan.

Robert Paget (an English immigrant and shipbuilder, according to Richard Saul Wurman's *Access Boston* guidebook, eighth edition) designed the original boats, which debuted in the Boston Public Garden in 1877. In the expansive history of the Swan Boats on its website, we learn that Paget drew his inspiration from Richard Wagner's opera *Lohengrin.* Today's versions are replicas, but the Paget family still runs the operation.

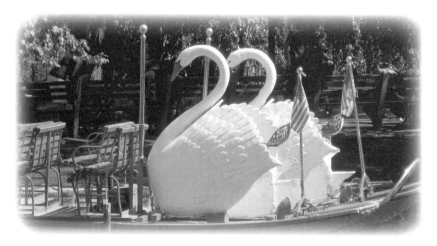

One of Boston's most beloved traditions

To increase the chances of optimal peacefulness, plan your visit for late afternoon on spring and fall weekdays or first thing in the morning in summer. Your best option is to choose a seat in the front row or to ride in the rear by the boatsman. As you float along with the real ducks and swans, take time to admire the Public Garden's extensive Victorian-inspired planting beds, with their colorful, exotic specimens. Be sure to look for turtles sunning themselves on the rocks near the lagoon's island. The Public Garden can be a birding hot spot during spring migration in May, so keep your ears peeled for unusual birdsong.

Once deposited back on land, wander along the Public Garden paths and admire the plantings close up. Even if you haven't brought a child with you, you'll want to stop by and visit Nancy Schön's beloved *Make Way for Ducklings* sculpture, depicting Mrs. Mallard and her eight babies. The once-secluded corner that's home to the magnificent *Angel of the Waters* by Daniel Chester French (most famous for the sculpture of President Abraham Lincoln at the Lincoln Memorial) is more open to traffic noise now that its yew hedges have been pruned down. But it's still my favorite place to sit and admire the beauty, both natural and man-made, of the Public Garden.

⌣ essentials

✉	Near the Charles Street entrance, between Boylston and Beacon streets, Boston, MA 02108
☎	(617) 522-1966
🌐	swanboats.com (Also visit schon.com for a photo of the enthralling ducklings sculpture, and chesterwood.org for more on the works of Daniel Chester French.)
$	**Adults:** $2.75; **seniors:** $2; **children ages 2–15:** $1.50
🕐	**Mid-April–June 20:** Daily, 10 a.m.–4 p.m. **June 21–Labor Day:** 10 a.m.–5 p.m. **Labor Day–the third Sunday in September:** Monday–Friday, noon–4 p.m.; Saturday–Sunday, 10 a.m.–4 p.m. *Note:* Boats cannot operate on rainy, windy, or extremely hot days.
🚊	**T:** Green Line, any train, to Arlington

peaceful place 112

TAVERN AT GRANITE LINKS GOLF CLUB
AT QUARRY HILLS

Quincy, MA (MAP ELEVEN)

CATEGORY ⌣ quiet tables ⭐

*Y*ou know that song "On a Clear Day You Can See Forever"? The lyricist must have been anticipating the Granite Links Golf Club. Though this was originally the site of the Quincy landfill, thanks to 8 million cubic yards of dirt from the urban tunnel excavation known as the Big Dig, it's now a hilltop with a 360-degree view. The vista sweeps from the South Shore, past the Blue Hills, over downtown Boston, to the North Shore, and out to the Harbor Islands.

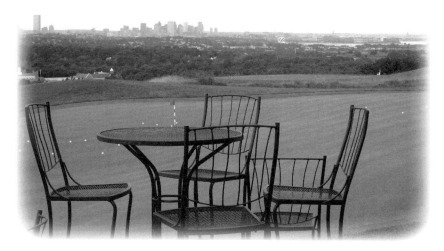

Panoramic views from this hilltop dining spot

Unless you're a golfer, Granite Links is one of the area's best-kept secrets for a visit. Luckily, non-duffers seeking a panorama and some quiet refreshment can usually find both. My suggestion is to pick an afternoon or early evening when it's warm enough to be outside—and clear enough for a great view—and head up the hill.

If you can get a table outside on the small balcony at the Tavern at Granite Links, you're in luck. (There are a few tables inside with great views, but I find the outdoor experience to be more serene.) If not, head over to the outdoor patio at the golf club's Crossing Nines Snack Shack patio and outdoor grill. It can be less tranquil there, especially on weekends, when there's live music; however, depending on your mood and the musical genre, it might just add to the relaxing atmosphere.

Either way—at the Tavern or at Crossing Nines—choose one of the wood-grilled pizzas and a glass of wine, and savor the natural beauty around you.

One tip: Crossing Nines is *the* place to be at sunset. On especially glorious evenings, you'll hear oohs and aahs of delight that won't disturb your inner calm as that magnificent orange orb disappears behind the gently rolling hills to the west.

↵ essentials

🖃   100 Quarry Hills Drive, Quincy, MA 02169

📞   (617) 689-1900, ext.112

🌐   granitelinksgolfclub.com

$ **Tavern entrées:** $10–$28; **Crossing Nines entrées:** $4–$10

🕐   Sunday–Thursday, 11 a.m.–10 p.m.; Friday–Saturday, 11 a.m.–11 p.m.

🚈   n/a

peaceful place 113

TOWER HILL BOTANIC GARDEN

Boylston, MA (MAP TWELVE)

CATEGORY ⌇ day trips & overnights ✪ ✪ ✪

*W*hile a botanic garden might seem like an unusual winter escape, Tower Hill is not your usual botanic garden. Indoors, you'll luxuriate in the scent of

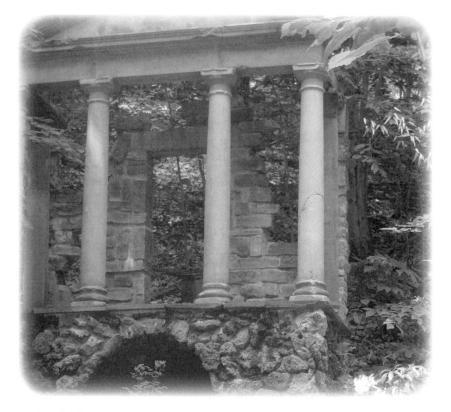

The Temple of Peace threshold to the Inner Park

lemons, limes, tangerines, and oranges. Palm trees, camellias, and other subtropical plants delight the eye. Outside, the woodland paths that are so charming in summer make serene places to cross-country ski or snowshoe in winter. Afterward, you can get a jump on spring by savoring the plant catalogs in the 8,000-volume library, or relax over some hot chocolate or soup at the garden's Twigs Café.

Of course, Tower Hill is an inviting haven in any season. Come spring, you'll be welcomed by flowering bulbs, birdsong, and apple blossoms. In summer, butterflies and extravagant blooms fill the garden. In fall, the vistas out across the valley to Mount Wachusett can be dazzling, especially from the Belvedere Outlook.

As the home of the Worcester County Horticultural Society, Tower Hill is serious about its plants. The Lawn Garden alone has hundreds of varieties of trees, shrubs, perennials, and ground covers, all nicely labeled for you. The Systematic Garden has plants organized by family. But there's also a whimsical side to Tower Hill that delights and refreshes the spirit.

Stroll through oak-lined Pliny's Allée to the fountain, which erupts at odd moments with a particularly impressive spout. Wander through the Inner Park to the enchanting Folly, Friendship Urn, and Temple of Peace, which capture the romantic spirit of 18th- and 19th-century landscaped parks. Children love the Wildlife Garden, where the "birdhouse" is really a screened-in viewing station for humans. At the nearby woodland pond, you'll see life-size statues of great blue herons; sometimes they're joined by the real thing.

Among my favorite Tower Hill spots are the breathtaking Moss Steps beneath the knolls beyond the Pan Statue and the fragrant Secret Garden off to the side of the pergolas. If you're walking the entire Loop Trail, the Rustic Pavilion overlooking the tranquil Wildlife Refuge Pond is a nice place to rest.

essentials

11 French Drive, Boylston, MA 01505   (508) 869-6111

towerhillbg.org (For an excellent orientation before you go—and to take along—click on "Distinctive Gardens" on the website home page; then hover over "Visit" and glide your mouse over to "Garden Map.")

$ Adults: $10; seniors: $7; children ages 6–18: $5; children age 5 and younger and members: free

Garden: Tuesday–Sunday and holiday Mondays, 9 a.m.–5 p.m. **Tour:** Sunday, 2 p.m.
Library: Tuesday, Thursday, and Saturday, 10 a.m.–4 p.m.
Twigs Café: Tuesday–Sunday and holiday Mondays, 11 a.m.–3 p.m. (with Tapas on the Terrace offered May–September: Wednesday, 4:30–7:30 p.m.)
Closed January 1, Thanksgiving, December 24–25, and December 31.

n/a

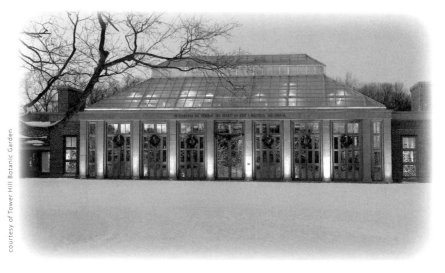

The garden's Orangerie in winter, a scene just an hour's drive west of Boston

courtesy of Tower Hill Botanic Garden

peaceful place 114

TRIDENT BOOKSELLERS & CAFÉ

Back Bay, Boston (MAP ONE)

CATEGORY ↝ shops & services ⭐

*W*here else can you walk through the door and be greeted by the aromas of both breakfast and incense? No doubt about it, the Trident is eclectic. Want to curl up with some obscure literary magazines from small independent colleges? Or perhaps you'd prefer to relax with a periodical on kick boxing or crystal healing? No matter how esoteric your interests, there's probably a magazine for you at Trident.

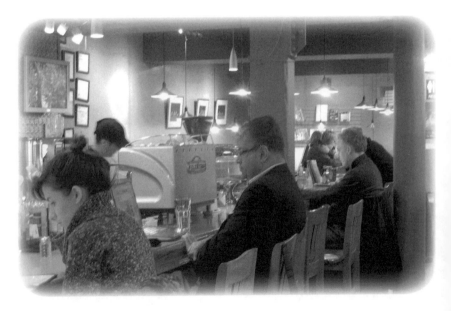

Taking a break at the bookstore café

The selection of books is similarly varied. Sure, there are best sellers on the shelves up front, but browse through the rest of the store, and you'll definitely find titles that you'd never see at the big chains.

Of course one of the attractions is the café itself. It's one of the rare places in Boston where you can linger over breakfast fare all day—and well into the night. And the lemon ricotta French toast is truly worthy of praise. There's also a great selection of menu items for vegetarians and vegans.

While the booths in the back offer a more tranquil space for reading or quiet conversation, I think that the tables in the windows up front provide a cozy place to use the free Wi-Fi, while enjoying the kind of people-watching that only Newbury Street can offer. Two distractions from complete peacefulness: Sometimes the music is loud and annoying— and weekend brunch can get crowded.

essentials

338 Newbury Street, Boston, MA 02115

(617) 267-8688

tridentbookscafe.com

Breakfast entrées (served all day): $2.50–$14.95; **lunch entrées:** $6.50–$13.95; **dinner entrées:** $13–$15

Daily, 8 a.m.–midnight

T: Green Line, B, C, or D train, to Hynes Auditorium

peaceful place 115

TRINITY CHURCH BOSTON, ORGAN CONCERTS

Back Bay, Boston (MAP ONE)

CATEGORY ↘ spiritual enclaves ✪ ✪ ✪

*I*n addition to having an exquisite pocket garden (see page 250), Trinity Church is one of Boston's—and, arguably, the world's—great architectural gems. According to the church website, renowned architect H. H. Richardson scrapped his original sketches that set forth a somewhat cookie-cutter Gothic Revival structure. Instead, using an unconventional Greek-cross plan, he designed chancel, nave, and transepts of equal size grouped around a central square. I wholeheartedly agree with the church's own description of the resulting edifice as a serene, yet massive, pyramid of space and light.

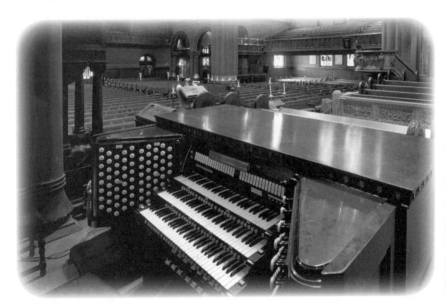

The weekly organ concerts: a heavenly escape

One of my favorite times to experience the calm of this majestic interior is at the Friday noontime organ concerts, when music lovers in the know make a pilgrimage to listen to works that range from Bach preludes and fugues to contemporary sacred music. As you gaze at the organist, it seems that he or she is performing on a single instrument. In reality, both the nave organ in the west wall of the church and the chancel organ in the altar area are being played at the same time, through a single console. With music in such a wide range of tone colors and effects surging out of 7,000 pipes, you feel the sound not just surrounding you, but also reverberating inside of you, no matter where you sit in the church.

At concert's end, instead of hurrying to the exit, take the opportunity to pause, close your eyes, and relax for a few minutes. Feeling refreshed and restored, you'll be ready for whatever the rest of your day or weekend may bring.

A gentle hint: Be sure to arrive in a timely fashion, as latecomers are seated only between musical selections.

↙ essentials

 206 Clarendon Street, Boston, MA 02116   (617) 536-0944

Concert schedule: trinitychurchboston.org/fridays-at-trinity
For details about Trinity's architecture, stained glass, and church tours: trinity churchboston.org (click on the boxed image "Learn about the Building and Its History")

$ **Concerts:** free, though suggested donation of $5. **Weekly Sunday tours:** free. **Guided and self-guided tours** (includes a map you can use for a path to other peaceful spots within these walls): Adults: $7; seniors and students: $5; children age 15 and younger accompanied by an adult: free

Friday concerts: first Friday in September–last Friday in June: 12:15 p.m.–1 p.m. **Visiting hours:** Monday, Friday, and Saturday, 9 a.m.–5 p.m.; Tuesday–Thursday, 9 a.m.–6 p.m.; Sunday, 1–6 p.m. **Self-guided tours:** Monday–Friday, 10 a.m.–3 p.m.; Saturday, 9 a.m.–4 p.m.; Sunday, 1–5 p.m. **Guided tours:** Times posted on website.

T: Green Line, any train, to Copley

peaceful place 116

TRINITY CHURCH BOSTON, ST. FRANCIS GARDEN

Back Bay, Boston (MAP ONE)

CATEGORY ⌣ urban surprises ✪ ✪

*I*t's not that this serene little garden is hard to find; it's just so out of sight that most people pass it by unknowingly. Located just a few steps from the corner of Clarendon and Boylston streets, one of the Back Bay's busiest intersections, Trinity Church's intimate St. Francis Garden is the quintessential secret urban refuge.

The sound of cascading water greets you as you approach this tiny outdoor space through the cloistered colonnade at the rear of the church. Then you see it, a compact,

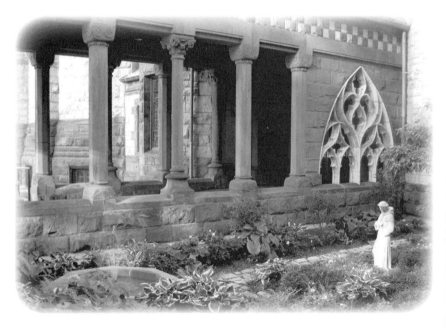

An inviting oasis in busy Copley Square

rectangular cobblestone-paved garden brimming with green and white: hostas, impatiens, roses, ferns, and small hydrangeas. Presiding over it all is a graceful statue of St. Francis.

Designed, planted, and cared for by members of the congregation and the church's facilities staff, this beautiful space has regularly been honored in the city's annual garden contest.

You cannot walk through the garden, but the surrounding wall is low enough to sit on, and the pillars provide an impromptu backrest. Listen to the fountain. Smile at the starlings or English sparrows splashing around in the birdbath (I once saw a hermit thrush here!). If you gaze through the portico to the west, you can watch the people hurrying across Copley Square and be glad that, for a few moments at least, you're not one of them.

⌣ essentials

🖃	206 Clarendon Street, Boston, MA 02116
☎	(617) 536-0944
🌐	trinitychurchboston.org
$	Free
🕐	Open 24/7
🚊	T: Green Line, any train, to Copley

peaceful place 117

UPSTAIRS ON THE SQUARE

Cambridge, MA (MAP SIX)

CATEGORY ◡ quiet tables ✪

*C*ome warm weather, my idea of dining heaven is an out-of-the way courtyard table with some dappled shade and a gentle breeze. Once Boston weather turns cold and gray, I yearn for a cozy space to dine by firelight. That's when I look for an opportunity to head to Harvard Square for a little R & R at Upstairs on the Square's Monday Club Bar.

Located—no surprise—up a flight of stairs, this is a funky space that makes me feel as though I've wandered into a party out of *Alice in Wonderland*. Bookended by ornate fire-places, the main room is a delight-ful mélange of purples, pinks, and greens, with animal prints and plaids thrown in for good measure. Off to the side, the Zebra Room presides as a sort of enclosed sun-porch, overlooking a tiny park. (Head up yet another staircase and you'll find the fancier Soirée Dining Room, also graced with two fireplaces, which bills itself as "reminiscent of a glowing and col-orful jewel-box-like supper club"— and that's no exaggeration.)

As you might expect, the most soothing time to experience the

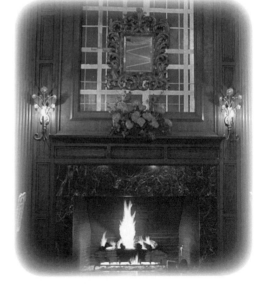

Dining by firelight in the Monday Club Bar

Monday Club Bar is between lunch and dinner service. Though the kitchen is closed then, you are welcome to linger over a glass of wine or a hot drink from the bar at one of the fireside tables overlooking Winthrop Street. For a tranquil late lunch or early supper during food-service hours, I prefer a table near the *rear* fireplace (particularly table L9).

I'm also fond of the Monday Club's Saturday afternoon tea. While the menu offers a choice of traditional teatime goodies, my preference is to order a little plate of the savory, light, and cheesy *gougères* and a kir royale. With a seat by the fireplace and a good friend (or a good book), it's the perfect escape.

⌣ essentials

⌑ 91 Winthrop Street, Cambridge, MA 02138

✆ (617) 864-1933

🌐 upstairsonthesquare.com

$ **Monday Club Bar and Zebra Room entrées:** Lunch: $10–$16; dinner: $10–$29; **Sunday brunch:** $14–$19; **afternoon tea:** $8–$35; **Soirée Dining Room entrées:** $15–$33

🕓 **Monday Club Bar and Zebra Room:** Daily, 11 a.m.–1 a.m. Lunch: Monday–Saturday, 11 a.m.–3 p.m. Dinner: Sunday–Thursday, 5–10 p.m.; Friday–Saturday, 5–11 p.m. **Brunch:** Sunday, 10 a.m.–3 p.m. **Afternoon tea:** Saturday, 2–4 p.m. (also on Sunday in the fall). **Soirée Dining Room:** Dinner: Tuesday–Thursday, 5–10 p.m.; Friday–Saturday, 5:30–11 p.m.

🚋 **T:** Red Line to Harvard

peaceful place 118

UPTOWN ESPRESSO CAFFE

South End, Boston (MAP FOUR)

CATEGORY ⌣ quiet tables 🟊 🟊

*I*f there was an Uptown Espresso Caffe in my neighborhood, I'd be there
every day. The walls in the cozy main room are a rainbow of calming colors—green,
lavender, and deep blue—and these hues provide a pleasant background for the rotating
gallery of works by local artists. The music is eclectic; the volume, pleasing.

When it's warm enough, you can sit outside on the tree-lined deck. And just about
any time is perfect for relaxing on the glass-enclosed sunporch. The coffees, lattes, and

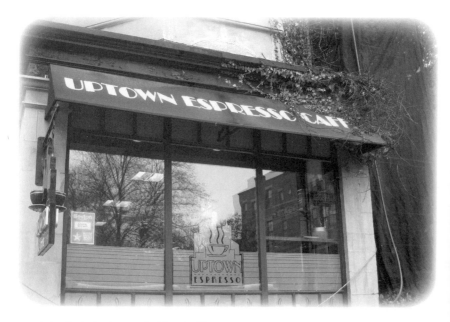

A favorite destination near the Mass Ave T

cappuccinos arrive table-side in big ceramic mugs that fit perfectly into your cupped hands. While the morning pastries and bagels are rather ordinary, the midday sandwiches and salads are made fresh and are noteworthy. There's also a wine list, in case you'd rather sip a glass of Pinot while reading your book in the late afternoon.

When I've been there, people are busy typing away on their laptops (no electricity, but free Wi-Fi). However, absolutely no one even dreams of talking on their cell phone. Peak hours on weekends can be a little busy, but other times, you can hear yourself think. Please, Uptown Espresso Caffe, open a branch in the Back Bay. Preferably near Fairfield Street.

essentials

☐ 563 Columbus Avenue, Boston, MA 02118

☎ (617) 236-8535

🌐 uptownespressoboston.com

$ **Coffee and tea:** $1.60–$4.45; **sandwiches, salads, and pizzas:** $5.25–$12

🕐 Monday–Thursday and Saturday, 7 a.m.–7 p.m.; Friday 7 a.m.–6 p.m.; Sunday, 8 a.m.–7 p.m.

🚇 **T:** Orange Line to Massachusetts Avenue Station

peaceful place 119

VILNA SHUL

Beacon Hill, Boston (MAP TWO)

CATEGORY ◡ spiritual enclaves ✪ ✪ ✪

he neighborhood is only 0.5 mile square in size, but in the late 19th century, Beacon Hill had a definite upstairs/downstairs aspect to it. On the south side were wealthy Brahmins with their stately Georgian-inspired townhouses and hidden gardens. On the other, known as the back side, were crowded tenements full of newly arrived immigrants, mostly Irish, Italian, and Eastern European Jews. Among the latter was a Lithuanian enclave called Anshei Vilner (the people of Vilnius). In 1919, they built a small synagogue that still stands today: the Vilna Shul, Boston's Center for Jewish Culture.

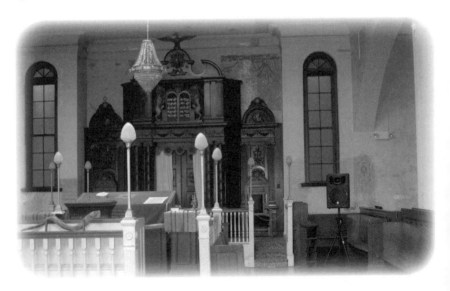

The sanctuary at the Vilna Shul

From the street, the building, with its large stained glass Star of David, is striking. An oft-repeated description of the Vilna Shul's interior is that while it is rooted in the design of medieval European synagogues, it evokes the simplicity of a Colonial New England meetinghouse. I couldn't agree more, and I think that's the source of its calming aura.

The first-floor museum presents an engaging history of the Jewish community in Boston. The upstairs sanctuary, with its vintage high-backed wooden pews and Star of David chandeliers, invites quiet contemplation. (I particularly like that, these days, I don't have to sit in the separate women's section, which is accessed through a stairway from the kitchen.) It's not uncommon for families of patients at nearby Massachusetts General Hospital to come here in search of spiritual uplift.

While I tend to think of the north side of Beacon Hill as being somewhat dark and shaded, the light streams through the sanctuary's skylight and the 12 large stained glass windows. Once a month, the Vilna Shul is the site of the lay-led, nondenominational Kabbalat Shabbat (Reception of the Sabbath) service. The synagogue also hosts lectures, movies, and concerts. Otherwise, unless there is a tour, you're more than likely to have the place to yourself.

essentials

18 Phillips Street, Boston, MA 02114

(617) 523-2324

vilnashul.org

$ Free, though donations suggested

Year-round: Wednesday, Thursday, and Friday, 11 a.m.–5 p.m. and by appointment
March 15–Thanksgiving: Sunday, 1–5 p.m.

T: Red Line to Charles/MGH

peaceful place 120

WELLESLEY COLLEGE BOTANIC GARDENS

Wellesley, MA (MAP NINE)

CATEGORY ⌣ parks & gardens ✪ ✪ ✪

*Y*ou don't have to be a budding botanist, or even a plant lover, to be completely enthralled by the experience of exploring the two gardens at Wellesley College, south of Boston. Whether you choose to wander up and down the small paths or over the swatches of lawn, there are pleasures for the senses at every turn at the Alexandra Botanic Garden and at the H. H. Hunnewell Arboretum.

When in bloom, the stands of flowering cherries, crab apples, and lilacs perfume their corners of the garden. The tiny waterfall between Cedar Knoll and the Viburnum Collection—another fragrant spot—delights the ears. And everywhere, in every season, you can behold the profusion of botanical rarities.

While a walk around Paramecium Pond can be most enjoyable, I happen to prefer the quiet of the Woodland Pond, with its marsh marigolds and horsetail rushes. (The latter are said to have provided Native Americans with both scouring powder and medicine.) Walk up the hill and spend a few moments contemplating the vista from the Margaret C. Ferguson memorial stone bench. As you pass the masses of rhododendrons so beloved by the arboretum's namesake, Mr. Hunnewell, keep in mind that it was H. H. himself who introduced this now ubiquitous species into the New England landscape.

Poetry lovers will enjoy reading the snippets of Robert Frost poems displayed here and there throughout the gardens in places appropriate to their themes. And on inclement days in the winter, the areas devoted to tropical and desert plants in the greenhouses—also, like the stone bench, named for Margaret C. Ferguson—will entice you.

✎ essentials

⌨   106 Central Street, Wellesley, MA 02481   ☎   (781) 283-3094

🌐   www.wellesley.edu/WCBG $ Free, though donations appreciated

🕐   **Outdoor gardens:** Daily, sunrise–sunset. **Greenhouses:** Daily, 8 a.m.–4 p.m.

🚌   n/a

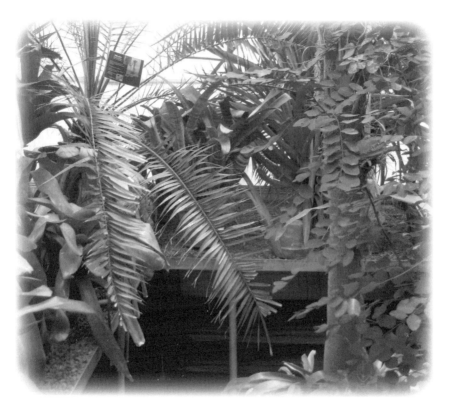

Greenery from exotic climes

peaceful place 121

WORLD'S END

Hingham, MA (MAP ELEVEN)

CATEGORY ↶ outdoor habitats ✪ ✪

*O*ne wonders if our planet might be a better place if the United Nations headquarters had been built here in the midst of this peaceful 251-acre coastal landscape. (Surprisingly, this bucolic place *was* on the short list of sites under consideration; perhaps the name World's End gave people pause.)

Had the United Nations materialized here, it's certain that those of us who appreciate tranquil pilgrimages to this site would be infinitely poorer. After all, where else can you find rolling hills, pastoral woodlands, butterfly-filled meadows, and saltwater

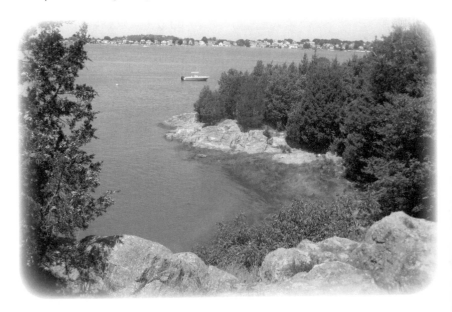

A peaceful little cove at World's End

marshes, plus a rocky granite coastline with sweeping views all the way to Boston, just 15 miles to the north?

None other than Frederick Law Olmsted designed the 4 miles of carriage paths for a 163-home community that, happily, never came to pass. Instead, the trails make strolling here such a sublime pleasure. Off these routes, myriad smaller trails lead to several unexpected vistas. You'll find that to be especially true in the far sections—on the Hingham Harbor side of the World's End peninsula and around Rocky Neck. If you're looking for cool woodlands with Boston views, head to the former; if you prefer more secluded coves, the latter is your best bet. The small loop off Weir River Road offers a quiet picnic spot with a view of the tidal marsh. (There's also an officially designated viewpoint off of Barnes Road.)

World's End is a lovely place to visit in any season, though the panoramas are most spectacular when the trees have shed their leaves. That's a little secret the fall-weekend foliage seekers don't know about. In fact, autumn is the busiest season: when the weather is nice, cars line up to get into the small parking area. Winter is the quietest season, and the carriage paths are wonderful for cross-country skiing or snowshoeing.

↵ essentials

📧	Martin's Lane, Hingham, MA 02043
📞	(781) 740-7233
🌐	thetrustees.org/places-to-visit/greater-boston/worlds-end.html
$	**Trustees, members, and children:** free; **nonmember adults:** $5
🕐	Daily, 8 a.m.–sunset
🚌	n/a

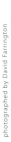

For nearly 40 years, Pennsylvania native Lynn Schweikart has nurtured an unabashed love affair with her adopted city of Boston. She loves wandering around its varied neighborhoods, returning to favorite haunts, and discovering new places.

A marketing communications specialist, writer, and brand storyteller, Schweikart has worked on high-profile accounts across a range of industries. She has been the recipient of numerous national and regional advertising creative awards. She also writes the blogs Savoring the Seasons and Peaceful Places Boston.

As someone who has spent her career in the high-pressure, fast-paced advertising world, Schweikart recognizes the restorative power that comes from moments of peacefulness and serenity. She enjoys travel, cooking, music, bird-watching, storytelling, kayaking, cheering on the Red Sox, and singing with the women's chorus Voices from the Heart. She's particularly fond of relaxing with her journal, camera, watercolors, and binoculars amid the marshes near Plum Island Sound—off the northeast coast of Massachusetts.

Schweikart holds a B. A. in sociology from Northwestern University. She divides her time between her homes in Boston and on the New Hampshire seacoast.